LANGUAGE CASE FILES IN NEUROLOGICAL DISORDERS

This book features case studies of ten individuals with acquired neurological disorders. These disorders have implications for speech, language, and communication, but to date they have not been the focus of research in speech-language pathology.

Chapters present a brief medical overview of each condition, followed by detailed linguistic analysis. A carefully assembled narrative captures the impact of each neurological disorder on an individual's daily life and social activities. This structured approach, supported by further reading and exercises, gives readers a nuanced understanding of each disorder's clinical presentation and language and communication features, and the complex interrelationship between language, communication, and cognitive and motor symptoms.

The book will be of interest to students of all levels, researchers, and clinicians in speech-language pathology and related disciplines, including neurology, psychiatry, and psychology.

Louise Cummings is Professor in the Department of English and Communication at The Hong Kong Polytechnic University. Her research interests within the field of speech-language pathology are pragmatic disorders, and language impairment in neurodegenerative disorders. In 2020, she published the volume *Language in Dementia*.

Routledge Research in Speech-Language Pathology
Series editor: Louise Cummings

Routledge Research in Speech-Language Pathology looks beyond traditional areas of study within the discipline to showcase topics historically underserved in research on communication disorders, highlighting fresh perspectives on issues of key importance in speech-language pathology. The series offers comprehensive treatments of communication disorders and the work of speech-language pathology with a view to pushing the field forward, critically examining challenges in addressing disparities in speech-language pathology and exploring the latest developments in related disciplines with implications for the future of research on communication disorders. Volumes in this series will be of particular interest to students, scholars and clinicians in speech-language pathology, speech and language therapy, and clinical linguistics, as well as related fields such as special education, psychology, neurology, psychiatry, social work and nursing.

Language Case Files in Neurological Disorders
Louise Cummings

For more information about this series, please visit: https://www.routledge.com/ Routledge-Research-on-Speech-Language-Pathology/book-series/RRSLP

LANGUAGE CASE FILES IN NEUROLOGICAL DISORDERS

Louise Cummings

Routledge
Taylor & Francis Group

NEW YORK AND LONDON

First published 2022
by Routledge
605 Third Avenue, New York, NY 10158

and by Routledge
2 Park Square, Milton Park, Abingdon, Oxon, OX14 4RN

Routledge is an imprint of the Taylor & Francis Group, an informa business

Library of Congress Cataloging-in-Publication Data
Names: Cummings, Louise, author.
Title: Language case files in neurological disorders / Louise Cummings.
Description: New York : Routledge, 2021. | Series: Routledge research in speech-language pathology | Includes bibliographical references and index.
Identifiers: LCCN 2021011301 | ISBN 9780367721282 (hardback) | ISBN 9780367721305 (paperback) | ISBN 9781003153559 (ebook)
Subjects: LCSH: Nervous system--Diseases--Case studies. | Language disorders--Case studies.
Classification: LCC RC359 .C86 2021 | DDC 616.8--dc23
LC record available at https://lccn.loc.gov/2021011301

ISBN: 978-0-367-72128-2 (hbk)
ISBN: 978-0-367-72130-5 (pbk)
ISBN: 978-1-003-15355-9 (ebk)

DOI: 10.4324/9781003153559

Typeset in Bembo
by SPi Technologies India Pvt Ltd (Straive)

CONTENTS

List of Figures and Tables   *vii*
Acknowledgements   *viii*

Introduction   1

Case Study 1: Corticobasal Degeneration   6

Case Study 2: Progressive Supranuclear Palsy   24

Case Study 3: Huntington's Disease   42

Case Study 4: Lewy Body Disease   60

Case Study 5: Multiple Sclerosis   82

Case Study 6: Parkinson's Disease   98

Case Study 7: Motor Neurone Disease   117

Case Study 8: Alcohol-Related Brain Damage   133

Case Study 9: Covid-19 Infection   155

Case Study 10: Guillain-Barré Syndrome   172

Conclusion   194

Glossary   *206*
Appendix   *233*
Index   *236*

FIGURES AND TABLES

Figures

4.1   Sample of Thomas' writing and copying spiral drawing,
      27 February 2018   63
4.2   Thomas' drawing of the wire cube in visuospatial abilities
      in ACE-R (scored 1 of 2)   65
A.1   Cookie Theft picture   234
A.2   Flowerpot Incident stimulus   235

Tables

1.1   Bob's speech sound errors   11
1.2   Cues used to elicit target words during confrontation naming   14
4.1   Thomas' range of symptoms according to his wife   64
10.1 Carly's performance across cognitive domains on
      neuropsychological evaluation   176

ACKNOWLEDGEMENTS

There are several people whose assistance I wish to acknowledge. I particularly want to thank Elysse Preposi, Editor, Routledge Research (US), for responding so positively to the proposal for this book. I am indebted to the individuals who participated in the PolyU language study. Their contribution and the assistance of their spouses and other family members have been invaluable in developing the case studies in this volume. I also wish to acknowledge the Faculty of Humanities of The Hong Kong Polytechnic University for its funding of this research through a start-up grant.

The following individuals assisted with participant recruitment to the PolyU language study and their support is gratefully acknowledged: Jimmy McClean (Ballymena and District Branch, Parkinson's UK); Sorcha McGuinness and Angie Smyth (Huntington's Disease Association of Northern Ireland); Kate Arkell (The PSP Association); Amelia Hursey (Parkinson's UK); and Patricia Forbes. Pro-Ed, Inc. has kindly given me permission to reproduce material.

Finally, I have been supported by family members and friends who are too numerous to mention individually. I am grateful to them for their kind words of encouragement during my many months of work on this volume.

INTRODUCTION

Like other health disciplines, speech-language pathology must continually reinvent itself to cope with new and emerging challenges. Nowhere is this reinvention more clearly seen than in the caseloads of **speech-language pathologists** (SLPs). Alongside clients with stroke- and trauma-induced **aphasia** and **dysarthria**, SLPs are now as likely to assess and treat individuals with adult-onset speech and language disorders related to neurodegenerative processes. While neurodegeneration related to **Alzheimer's disease** has been extensively studied, many other neurodegenerative processes are still poorly understood. They include disorders such as **Lewy body disease** and **corticobasal degeneration**, to name but two. Where disorders like **Parkinson's disease** and **multiple sclerosis** were once thought to have implications only for speech production, there is now growing recognition that clients with these disorders also often present with complex, high-level language impairments even in the absence of **dementia**. The cognitive basis of many of these impairments, their 'masking' by motor and other symptoms, and the prioritisation of clients' physical health needs (e.g. nutrition) by healthcare providers have often resulted in the neglect of language in individuals with **neurodegenerative disorders** and the treatment of only speech production and swallowing problems. SLPs can, and should, address the language impairments of these clients. The case studies in this book are an attempt to do just that.

The case studies in this book examine language in adults with different types of neurodegeneration. Adult-onset neurodegeneration is typically associated with ageing. The **prevalence** rates of **Parkinson's disease**, for example, almost double with every five-year interval between 50 and 69 years of age for both men and women.[1] However, neurodegeneration is also a consequence of the toxic effects of long-term alcohol consumption on the brain and infectious diseases

DOI: 10.4324/9781003153559-1

such as SARS-CoV-2, the virus that is responsible for the Covid-19 pandemic. But while age-related neurodegeneration and its sequelae have been extensively characterised, much less research effort has been directed towards understanding neurodegeneration in the context of alcoholism and infectious diseases. Adults with language disorders related to neurodegeneration arising from alcohol abuse are noticeable by their absence in speech-language pathology. These clients are not in the caseloads of SLPs or the focus of research studies. This omission cannot be justified on grounds of prevalence. With an estimated 35% of those with alcohol dependence exhibiting post-mortem evidence of **alcohol-related brain damage** (ARBD),[2] the prevalence of ARBD exceeds that of many more widely recognised neurodegenerative disorders. This omission also cannot be justified by a lack of clinical need. As the case studies of this volume illustrate, individuals with ARBD can experience significant language and communication problems. Social stigma and exclusion explain the lack of priority afforded to these individuals in speech-language pathology. SLPs can, and should, address this exclusion by assessing and treating the language impairments of these clients.

Accordingly, the motivation for this volume is two-fold. First, it is to encourage SLPs to take a broader view of the impairments that they can assess and treat in adults with neurodegenerative disorders. Certainly, **motor speech disorders** (e.g. dysarthria and **apraxia of speech**) and swallowing problems continue to require assessment and treatment by SLPs. But consideration must also be given to impairments of language, an area that has been somewhat overlooked by clinicians. Second, it is to encourage SLPs to address a much wider range of neurodegenerative disorders than has been considered in clinical practice and research to date. These disorders include conditions like Lewy body disease that are still poorly understood and recognised. They also include conditions like ARBD that have been neglected on account of the social stigma and exclusion experienced by individuals with addiction problems. These disorders are among the new health challenges that SLPs must address. In order to adapt their clinical practice to meet these challenges, SLPs must first be able to characterise language in these neurodegenerative disorders. This book is an important first step in this direction.

From the outset, it is important to say something about the case-study approach that is adopted in this volume. Case studies have had something of a bad press. They are often criticised for their apparent lack of scientific rigour and poor generalisation: "Case study research has sometimes been criticised for lacking scientific rigour and providing little basis for generalisation (i.e. producing findings that may be transferable to other settings)".[3] Clearly, it is not intended that readers should be able to infer that every individual who has Parkinson's disease or Lewy body disease will have the same presentation as the individuals with these conditions featured in the case studies in this volume. But this is not a weakness of the case-study approach adopted in this book. It is a fact that no two people with any neurodegenerative disease will have the same presentation. The unique manifestation of these disorders in each person who has them is exactly what a case study is ideally suited to capture. Moreover, case studies allow readers to see the complex interrelation-ships that exist between language and communication, and an individual's social functioning, activities of daily living and much else besides. The complex interplay between these factors is all but completely occluded from view in experimental studies of people with neurodegenerative disorders. The case-study approach is a powerful research method when the aim is to characterise complex disorders that are variously manifested in the naturalistic contexts in which they occur.

The case-study approach has several other advantages. Any study of language has greater ecological validity when it is conducted in the real-life contexts in which language unfolds. This includes the use of language to relate stories to others, to engage in conversation, and to describe simple routines and events in the world around us. An examination of language in these contexts requires detailed, qualitative analysis to understand the nature and source of any break-down. Case studies are a sensitive means through which to explore these different types of language use. Analysis of extended extracts of language can be under-taken, with comparisons possible across several potentially interesting parameters. These parameters include the presence of an interlocutor in conversation versus the absence of an interlocutor in narration. They also include the influence of a familiar script and pictorial support on story retell versus story retell of novel material that is presented auditorily only. Case studies permit an examination of language across all modalities and contexts to a level of detail that is unmatched by other research methods. This is a major impetus for the case-study approach that is adopted in this volume.

To counter criticisms of case studies, it will be shown that the case studies in this book can be used to address several significant questions. They include:

- To what extent are impairments of language in adults with neurodegenera-tive disorders related to deficits in linguistic structure?
- To what extent are impairments of language in adults with neurodegenera-tive disorders related to diagnosed or self-reported cognitive deficits?
- Are language impairments present in adults with neurodegenerative disor-ders even in the absence of dementia or cognitive impairment?
- Are adults with neurodegenerative disorders adept at compensating for their speech and language impairments?
- Do impaired and preserved language skills co-exist, even within the same level of language?
- Do adults with neurodegenerative disorders exhibit impairments of linguis-tic competence, communicative competence, or both?
- Do conversational partners facilitate or dominate exchanges with adults who have neurodegenerative disorders?

Based on the case studies presented here, these questions will be addressed in the conclusion of the volume. The answers will touch on issues such as the interface between language and cognition, the level of integration or modularity of different aspects of language, the components of language most vulnerable to neurodegeneration, and the consequences for social communication of language impairment related to neurodegeneration. These are important issues which the case-study approach can help us answer.

Finally, it is worth saying a few words about the format adopted in each of the case studies. Each study begins with a *Key Facts and Figures* section. This section presents information on the prevalence and **incidence (epidemiology)** and medical causes and risk factors (**aetiology**) of each neurodegenerative disorder. The age of onset, sex ratio, survival time and symptoms are also addressed in this section. The aim is to provide a brief, accessible introduction to the medical aspects of each neurodegenerative disorder for readers from diverse disciplinary backgrounds. In the *Background* section, the individual at the centre of the case study is introduced. This section discusses the family background, employment history and date of diagnosis of the person with a neurodegenerative disorder. Many of the individuals featured in these case studies have taken years to arrive at a definitive diagnosis of their condition. This long and difficult journey is charted in this section, along with various medical investigations and consultations conducted along the way. In *Clinical Symptoms*, the full range of symptoms experienced by the individual with neurodegenerative disorder are presented. This section includes motor, sensory, cognitive and psychiatric symptoms. It also includes gastro-intestinal problems, swallowing difficulties and sleep disorders that can impact adversely on an individual's quality of life. Motor and cognitive symptoms can have significant implications for language and communication. Motor dysfunction, for example, may restrict the use of **gesture** in communication.

The section *Daily Activities* explores the impact of a person's neurodegenerative disorder on the routines and activities of daily life, including an individual's social networks, leisure pursuits and personal care activities. As well as the loss of activities (e.g. loss of friendship networks), this section also discusses the activities that a person with neurodegenerative disorder is successful in maintaining as well as new activities (e.g. participation in a support group) that may have arisen since diagnosis. Most individuals featured in the case studies are on complex drug regimens, not only for the control of their symptoms but also for the treatment of co-morbidities such as high blood pressure. In the section *Medication*, these drugs, their doses and any side-effects for the person with neurodegenerative disorder are outlined. The central focus of each case study is on the implications of a neurodegenerative disorder for a person's speech, language and communication skills. In the *Communication* section, a detailed analysis of language is undertaken, from **phonology**, **morphology** and **syntax** to **vocabulary**, **semantics**, **pragmatics** and **discourse**. Linguistic analysis is conducted on extended language samples recorded by the author during visits to participants' homes or during online meetings, with examples presented for illustration. A detailed summary of language skills and impairments is presented in the section *Communication Profile* at the end of each case study.

Finally, readers are supported in their learning by several additional sections and features in each study. Annotated readings are included under *Suggestions for Further Reading*. Most recommended readings examine language in further detail. A smaller number provide readers with a medical overview of a neurodegenerative disorder. Each is chosen for its accessibility to readers from different disciplinary backgrounds. At the end of each chapter are *Questions* and *Answers* sections. Questions encourage readers to develop practical skills of language analysis, using data from the transcribed audio-recording of the person with neurodegenerative disorder. These exercises have a dual purpose. They ease the load on time-pressed instructors who have a set of prepared exercises for use in class and as homework activities. Also, students can use these exercises and the answers to them for self-study and revision purposes. Lastly, a detailed glossary of all key terms used in the case studies appears at the end of the volume. The glossary terms correspond to words in bold type in the main text. The glossary removes the need for readers to consult other sources to find definitions of key terms and allows the book to stand as a self-contained resource.

References

[1] Parkinson's UK (2017) *The Incidence and Prevalence of Parkinson's in the UK: Results from the Clinical Practice Research Datalink Reference Report*. London: Author.
[2] Royal College of Psychiatrists (2014) *Alcohol and Brain Damage in Adults with Reference to High-Risk Groups*. London: Author.
[3] Crowe, S., Cresswell, K., Robertson, A., Huby, G., Avery, A. and Sheikh, A. (2011) 'The case study approach', *BMC Medical Research Methodology*, 11: 100. http://www. biomedcentral.com/1471-2288/11/100.

CASE STUDY 1

Corticobasal Degeneration

KEY FACTS AND FIGURES:

- Corticobasal degeneration (CBD) is a tauopathy in which there is deposition of abnormal tau protein in the brain. Corticobasal syndrome (CBS), the most common phenotype, is characterised by asymmetric rigidity and apraxia, cortical sensory deficits, dystonia and myoclonus. Patients with clinical CBD can have non-CBD pathology such as Alzheimer's pathology.[1]
- The prevalence of CBD is 10.84 per 100,000 and the incidence is 1.61 per 100,000. These figures are based on a population of 1.69 million in Cambridgeshire and Norfolk in England. A crude prevalence of 9 per 100,000 is reported in a rural district in Japan. The age-standardised incidence rate is 0.02 per 100,000/year in a Russian population-based study.[2-4]
- Age at onset and survival time in CBD have been reported in several studies. In a review of 267 nonoverlapping pathologically confirmed CBD cases from published reports and brain banks, mean age at symptom onset was 63.7 years (range 45–77.2 years) and mean disease duration was 6.6 years (range 2.0–12.5 years).[5]
- Motor, behavioural, cognitive and language symptoms are common in CBD. In one clinical sample of 48 patients with CBD, apraxia (93.8%) was the most common symptom followed by behavioural changes (75%), rigidity (68.8%), postural instability (66.7%), language impairment (66.7%), akinesia (62.5%), dystonia (54.2%) and supranuclear gaze paresis (45.8%).[2]

DOI: 10.4324/9781003153559-2

- Speech, language and cognitive impairments are common in CBD. In a clinical sample of 33 patients with CBS, motor speech disorder was present in 33%, agrammatism in 48% and sentence comprehension problems in 60%. Impairments of executive functions were reported in 81% of the sample.[6] Language disturbances in some patients with CBD manifest as an aphasia syndrome.[7]
- CBD is a challenging disorder to diagnose. It can present with multiple phenotypes, and other neurodegenerative disorders with a different underlying pathology can mimic its clinical course.[8]

Background

Bob (not his real name) is a man of 66; 4 years who was diagnosed with corticobasal degeneration (CBD) in September 2017. [Bob passed away on 25 March 2021. He was last seen in clinic by his neurologist on 10 February 2021, following which his diagnosis was revised to "progressive non-fluent aphasia – corticobasal syndrome".] He is a former joiner. His wife is a retired science teacher. Both have children from previous relationships. Bob's wife noticed some changes in him a few years ago that "started alarm bells ringing". In August 2014, some guests at a family wedding expressed concerns for Bob as he did not seem to be himself. Shortly afterwards, his wife noticed that he was experiencing difficulties with **coordination**. In the third week of August 2014, Bob and his wife were walking along the promenade in their hometown. Bob went to put his mobile phone in his pocket but completely missed his pocket and ended up kicking the phone ahead of him. A couple of weeks after this incident, Bob's wife noticed that he was unable to help her change the duvet on the bed, a task he had completed many times before. Bob was unable to bring the duvet and cover together and eventually had to abandon the task. Not long after this, Bob's wife noticed that he was unable to coordinate actions such as getting dressed and putting on his shoes. Bob sat and looked at his shoes as if he were lost. By August 2016, Bob was unable to measure and cut pieces of wood to a required length, something he had done since he was 14 years old. Bob has no family history of **dementia** or mental illness.

There ensued a long-running series of medical and cognitive investigations to establish the cause of Bob's difficulties. In November 2014, Bob was referred for an MRI of the head. He had experienced right-sided facial weakness and speech difficulty about two months earlier. His general practitioner had referred him for a **CT scan**, but no abnormality was detected. Bob presented with bilateral upgoing plantars without any sensory loss. He had expressionless facies but no other signs of **Parkinson's disease**. The MRI was undertaken to investigate if there was any **ischaemia** or other diagnosis that might explain his symptoms. An MRI was conducted on 2 December 2014, but it did not identify any acute intracranial abnormality. On 6 August 2015, Bob was assessed on the Folstein Mini-Mental State Examination. He scored 28/30, indicating no/minimal cognitive impairment. This assessment was repeated on 26 May 2016. Bob scored 27/30 on this occasion.

After further deterioration of Bob's cognitive abilities and other skills, he underwent a psychiatric assessment in July 2016. His wife reported **memory** problems and communication difficulties, including word-finding problems and **stuttering**. Bob had lost his job in May 2016 and had been feeling low. He was prescribed an antidepressant, Citalopram 20 mg, which improved his memory slightly although further deterioration continued. His wife also reported that his judgement was impaired, leading him to cross the road recklessly and do risky things at home. Bob often lost his way and walked off without telling anyone. He liked to joke about the mistakes he was making and was not aware of the deterioration in his cognitive function. Bob's speech was observed to be monotonous, slow and stuttering. His mood was euthymic. There was no evidence of psychotic features and no thoughts of self-harm or harming others. The Mini-Mental State Examination was conducted, and Bob again scored 27/30 (no/minimal cognitive impairment). The plan for Bob's continued care included a referral to the Memory Service on 26 July 2016.

Bob was seen at the Memory Service a short time after referral. A report by the Memory Service on 1 November 2016 indicated that he was assessed on the Addenbrooke's Cognitive Examination Revised (ACE-R). He displayed cognitive impairment across all domains, but most notably in tasks of **attention**, language and memory. Bob underwent further neuropsychological assessment on three occasions during January 2017. He was assessed on the Wechsler Memory Scale Fourth Edition (WMS IV), the Wechsler Adult Intelligence Scale Fourth Edition (WAIS IV), items from the Delis Kaplan Executive Function System (DKEFS), the Boston Naming Test (BNT), and the Pyramids and Palm Trees Test (PPTT). Bob's premorbid intellectual function had not been assessed but was assumed to be in the 'average' range. His current intellectual function, as assessed on the WAIS IV, was in the 'extremely low' range, suggesting a significant decline. Bob displayed slowed processing across a range of tests. However, when given time to complete tasks, his ability was often preserved. His motor speed was slow.

Bob's performance on memory tasks displayed some inconsistencies. On some tests of **short-term memory** and **working memory**, he demonstrated impairment. Bob also required repetition of instructions. His verbal memory ability on the WMS IV was in the 'average' range. Bob's visual memory fell within the 'borderline range' (lower limits) and was a weakness relative to his verbal memory. Bob's visuospatial constructional abilities were intact. On tasks of **executive function**, he demonstrated preserved ability to sequence information but had difficulty switching attention. On tasks of **verbal fluency**, Bob's performance fell within the 'impaired' range. His performance was negatively impacted by his slowed speed of information processing. Bob displayed marked word-finding difficulties during a **confrontation naming** task. His main errors were phonemic in nature and failure to retrieve the word. He made no semantic errors and his object recognition appeared intact. In her conclusions, the neuropsychologist remarked that Bob's most pervasive difficulty was severe **psychomotor slowing** which had downstream effects on all other domains tested. Bob's short-term memory impairments also compromised his ability to encode information on some subtests, while Bob also displayed difficulties in some tasks assessing executive function (verbal fluency, arithmetic and switching).

In September 2017, Bob was examined by a consultant neurologist at a regional hospital. Bob had previously been examined by a neurologist whom he had consulted privately. The consultant neurologist reported reduced facial expression and somewhat mumbling speech with obvious word-finding difficulties. There was no **tremor**. Bob's blood pressure was 120/65 (normal) with no postural drop. Bob had severe difficulty performing rapid alternating movements with his tongue and hands and he could not copy hand gestures at all. He had full power in the limbs and normal eye movements. Tone was slightly increased in the lower limbs, but it was normal in the upper limbs. The plantars were flexor. Bob's coordination was a little hesitant in the lower limbs. He walked with a slight stoop, but his stride length was reasonably normal. His posture was generally rigid throughout. Bob had severe difficulties trying to copy a simple geometric shape. The neurologist reviewed Bob's brain imaging. His PET scan showed some areas of **hypometabolism**, and there was evidence of **atrophy** over the **parietal lobes** on MRI and CT. The neurologist confirmed a diagnosis of CBD, a suspicion of the neurologist whom Bob had seen privately, and recommended follow-up in 6 months.

Clinical Symptoms

On first encounter with the author, Bob's wife reports that his gross and **fine motor movements** are compromised. He walks with a shuffling gait which, she says, was worse at the start of the disease. His movement has become so slowed that his wife reports that it is like "watching someone in very slow motion". He is no longer able to make fast, spontaneous movements. The left side of Bob's body is very stiff. He experiences deadness in his left arm which his wife remarks "does not do what he wants it to do". She states that he frequently "forgets" about it. There are intermittent jerks in his arms and legs even as he sleeps. There are no reports of increased falls. Bob's fine motor movements are very restricted. He cannot do up a button or tie his shoe laces. He can only eat with one hand.

Bob's wife reports that he now engages in less conversation (i.e. initiating and maintaining) and has become increasingly socially withdrawn. Bob has experienced deterioration in his swallow, resulting in increased saliva build-up and **drooling**. There have also been a few instances when he has laughed out loud while he is fast asleep. His wife reports that he is sometimes "too smiley" which his neurologist has said is part of the condition. Bob experiences significantly increased lethargy. He takes naps during the day and goes to bed at around 7.30 p.m. There has been no change to his personality in terms of irritability or agitation.

Daily Activities

All of Bob's daily activities have been negatively affected by CBD. He cannot make plans and follow them through to fruition. He cannot follow simple instructions to help with the housework. He is unable to plan how to cook a meal and cannot use the cooker safely. Although he was formerly a joiner, his wife reports that he now has no idea how to measure using a ruler. He is still able to empty the dishwasher every morning. All aspects of Bob's personal care are affected by his condition. He cannot shave or wash his teeth and has difficulty with personal hygiene when he uses the toilet. He needs help with showering as he does not know where the water is. He cannot dress himself. Because he is very stiff, he finds it difficult to take off clothes especially trousers and so he needs help undressing. It takes Bob twice as long to finish a meal. Bob attends a vocational and leisure rehabilitation centre in a nearby town 2.5 days per week. He is also attending occupational therapy for 2.5 days a week and "loves it", according to his wife.

Medication

Previously, Bob took Sinemet 62.5 mg (two tablets three times daily) and Memantine 20 mg daily. However, these drugs produced little positive response and so Bob's neurologist recommended discontinuing them. Sinemet is a combination of carbidopa and **levodopa** for the treatment of Parkinson's disease and syndrome. Memantine is used to slow the neurotoxicity involved in **Alzheimer's disease** and other neurodegenerative diseases.

Communication

The earliest sign of communication difficulties was that Bob noticed he was having difficulty finding words. Although his wife reports that he communicates "reasonably well", she nonetheless acknowledges many areas of impaired communication. She describes Bob as speaking in monosyllables using a low-pitched voice that has little **intonation**. His cheeks and mouth sometimes give a jerk that upsets the flow of his speech. He does not initiate conversation at all, but he can answer questions and engage to a certain extent. His wife reports that at times his talking "doesn't fully make sense". Bob has almost fully lost his ability to write, even when he is asked to copy written words. He can still read but loses concentration very quickly. Bob received speech and language therapy about a year ago.

The author visited Bob and his wife on the afternoon of 31 July 2018. An audio-recording was made as Bob completed several language tasks in the kitchen of their home. Bob was friendly, responsive and participated cooperatively in all activities. He displayed **impulsivity**, a common feature in CBD.[9] He began producing words in a timed task before the author had completed the task instructions. When walking with the author back to the train station after the test session, Bob abruptly left her side and darted into a shop. Although Bob's production of speech sounds was clear on many occasions, there were numerous islands of unintelligible speech during the session. Bob spoke very quietly and had to be repeatedly reminded to increase his volume "for the benefit of the recording". He was able to understand questions posed to him during conversation and follow instructions to each task, although comprehension of task instructions was undoubtedly facilitated by the reformulations provided as standard by the author. Bob made appropriate use of **humour** and laughter throughout the interaction. One instance occurred when he remarked that he did not know what his favourite TV programme was because his wife always had the controls and turned the television onto something else.

An examination of the language sample that was recorded revealed Bob made numerous speech sound errors (see Table 1.1). Phonological and apraxic speech errors have been previously reported in patients with CBD.[10,11,12] Bob displayed these errors across six different contexts: spontaneous conversation; immediate story recall; sentence generation; **semantic fluency**; confrontation naming; and Cinderella narration. Some of Bob's errors displayed the inconsistency of apraxic speech errors (e.g. 'sheep' → [ʃɪp] [ʃeɪp] [ʃip]). Other errors involved sound substitutions

TABLE 1.1 Bob's speech sound errors

Spontaneous conversation	Immediate story recall
'joiner' → [dʒɪmə] [dʒɪgəmə]	'people' → [pʌli]
'started' → [staktɪt]	'barn' → [har]
'Donegal' → [dʌnɪdɔl]	
'Thursday' → [əɜrədeɪ]	
'understand' → [ʌndərstɛsɪn]	
Sentence generation	**Semantic fluency**
'leaves' → [leɪvz]	'sheep' → [ʃɪp] [ʃeɪp] [ʃip]
'hospital' → [hɔstəbɪl]	'cat' → [hat]
Confrontation naming	**Cinderella narration**
'duck' → [dʌs]	'shoe' → [ʃɒp]
'emu' → [ju]	
'pumpkin' → [pʌmpʌm]	
'accordion' → [əkɜri] [aɪron]	
'thimble' → [əɪndɪl]	
'seahorse' → [hɔrs haʊs (.) si sɔr]	

(e.g. 'duck' → [dʌs]), syllable deletions (e.g. 'emu' → [ju]), sound omissions (e.g. 'barn' → [har]), and sound transpositions (e.g. 'hospital' → [hɔstəbɪl]).

Dysfluency is reported in CBD.[13] Bob's **fluency** was occasionally disrupted by syllable and word repetition:

> I stacked [started] su su su su su su seventeen
> I always held a, a, a, a, a, an eye of me ear all my working time
> and it's in, in, in every morning in

Agrammatism is a feature of expressive language in CBD.[13] Bob's expressive **syntax** was quite limited. Occasionally, he produced utterances that were well-formed including the following examples in which **clauses** are linked by means of **coordination** and **subordination**:

> I like going to the boys down in the golf, <u>but</u> I haven't been down for a while
> don't know <u>because</u> it's always turned on to something else
> he said to me (.) <u>that</u> I'd have to come again

Often, however, he omitted words from sentences or abandoned sentences midway, as in the following examples:

> we […] up to the doctor's place
>
> > *(omission of main verb)*

> he […] going to get
>
> > *(omission of auxiliary verb)*

> I am (.) because (.) most of them didn't understand
>
> > *(abandoned sentence)*

Although Bob's understanding of complex questions in conversation was adequate for the most part, there were occasional difficulties with comprehension such as in the following exchange between the author (INV) and Bob:

INV: so, what was it that nearly killed you?
BOB: eh (1:39) yes it did

Even when speakers with CBD can pass grammatical comprehension tasks, they have still been found to have impairments of syntactic knowledge, evidenced by selective deficits in detecting violations in verb–**subject** agreement, interrogatives and clitic movement.[14]

Bob's lexical-semantic abilities were also examined. Occasionally, he produced semantic errors during the language tasks, such as the following error that arose during sentence generation. Bob had previously worked as a joiner and kept a pencil for making measurements behind his ear. When asked to produce a sentence that contained the word *pencil*, he used the semantically related word *eye* before producing *ear*, with the target word *pencil* omitted altogether:

I always held a, a, a, a, a, a, an <u>eye</u> of me <u>ear</u> all my working time (.) life

Other semantic errors occurred during the Cookie Theft picture description task (see Appendix). Bob produced words that are semantically related to the target words on the left of the arrows below:

mother's making (.) the dishes

(*washing* → *making*)

he's going to break his head

(*hit* → *break*)

cookies in a box

(*jar* → *box*)

Several of Bob's semantic errors involved action verbs. In CBD, action verb naming is impaired and is more impaired than object naming, a deficit that is related to degeneration of the fronto-parietal-subcortical circuits involved in action knowledge and action representation.[15,16]

Bob completed semantic fluency, a test of lexical knowledge and retrieval ability. He obtained a score of six animal names in 60 seconds. Although this score is low relative to healthy subjects, it is consistent with semantic fluency scores reported for individuals with CBD in the literature. In one study, patients with CBD obtained an average semantic fluency score for eight categories of 43.3 words (or 5.4 words for a single category in 60 seconds), while healthy subjects achieved an average of 113.7 words for eight categories (or 14.2 words for a single category in 60 seconds).[10] Bob also completed **phonemic fluency** which assesses **lexical retrieval** and executive function skills. He produced seven words beginning with the letter 'F' in 60 seconds. This is low relative to healthy controls who can produce 44.6 words for the letters F, A, S combined (or 14.9 words for each letter in 60 seconds). However, it is higher than phonemic fluency scores for individuals with CBD reported in the literature (10 words for the letters F, A, S combined or 3.3 words for each letter in 60 seconds).[10] Bob's phonemic fluency score raises the possibility that executive function skills such as **inhibition** are impaired in addition to lexical search and retrieval.

TABLE 1.2 Cues used to elicit target words during confrontation naming

Semantic and phonemic cue

ostrich → "it's a bird with big long legs, it's a big tall neck, lays very large eggs, it's an ost, ost"

pineapple → "this is something you can eat, it's very sweet, it's a nice sweet taste, it's, it's you can get it in tins as well but I'm sure it's nicer if you buy it fresh, um hum it's a pie, pine"

pumpkin → "you can carve bits of it out in Halloween can't you it's a pump"

Semantic, gestural and phonemic cue

accordion → "this is a it's a type of musical instrument and you play it if, if you move your hands in and out don't you your arms and hands in and out (*gestures*) it's an it sounds ah core"

lobster → "lives in the in the sea doesn't it and it's got these big (*gestures pincers*) [P: *you have to put it in alive which is*] you do it's not so nice it's not having to do that you plonk it into the boiling water don't you un hum lob, lob, lobs"

Semantic, orthographic and phonemic cue

spanner → "this is something a car mechanic might use … if you're trying to tighten up nuts on something … begins with an 'S' spa"

During confrontation naming, Bob was only able to name 10 of 18 pictures accurately and without the use of cues by the author. A range of cues were required to elicit target words for the remaining eight pictures. These involved a combination of semantic, phonemic, gestural and orthographic cues (see Table 1.2).

It is interesting to note that even as Bob was unable to name certain pictures, he was able to contribute to the cuing strategies that the author used to elicit his production of target words. This occurred during naming of *pumpkin, lobster* and *spanner*. It indicated that Bob still retained considerable knowledge about the target word and its meaning even though he was unable to retrieve its name from his mental lexicon:

PUMPKIN: "you can put it out in (.) in Halloween"
LOBSTER: "you have to put it in alive which is ahh it's pretty messy"
SPANNER: "or taking them [nuts] off"

Alongside lexical retrieval deficits in confrontation naming, Bob exhibited **word-finding difficulty** in conversation with the author (INV) and his wife (PAR), as illustrated below:

BOB: and (.) then (.) we had to do a couple ah (1:26) we up to the doctor's place in Coleraine
INV: um hum
BOB: we had to do two what would you call it?
PAR: talks
BOB: talk

Word-finding difficulty is a feature of language in CBD.[13] It was noted by Bob's wife in July 2016, two years before the author's visit. Bob quite commonly displayed markers of word-finding difficulty, including the use of timed pauses and micro-pauses especially before **content words**, the presence of **fillers** like *ah* and *um*, and questions to his wife such as *what would you call it?* **Circumlocutions** were also present and were further evidence that Bob had a word-finding difficulty:

Sam and Fred story:

> the weather come down
>
> > (used to express *it was raining*)

Cookie Theft picture description:

> he's put them down
>
> > (used to express *he passed the cookies to the girl*)

Bob displayed many intact aspects of **pragmatics**. He was able to take turns in conversation and contributed relevant, mostly informative utterances. As mentioned above, he used **humour** and laughter appropriately during the session. There was evidence that he had retained some idiomatic uses of language such as when he said that he was "last out in the grass" to describe his retirement (**idiom**: *put somebody out to pasture*). Bob also understood the author when she said, "so somebody else <u>calls the shots</u> when it comes to the TV programmes". Bob was able to repair conversational misunderstanding on the part of the author. When the author asked Bob what his favourite TV programme was, he responded that he did not know "because it's always turned on to something else". The author then attempted to check her understanding of what Bob had said by stating "you always turn it onto something else". At that point, Bob corrected the author's misunderstanding by saying that somebody else (namely, his wife) did:

INV: what's your favourite television programme?
BOB: don't know because it's always turned on to something else
INV: oh, you always turn it on to something else
BOB: no, somebody else or (2:16) takes it ah

There is, however, some limited evidence of pragmatic and **discourse** difficulties in speakers with CBD. In a case study, a woman with CBD produced only 38% appropriate items on the Pragmatic Protocol,[17] with impairments recorded in **topic management**, **turn taking**, lexical selection/use (i.e. specificity and accuracy), and **cohesion** of comments.[12] During narrative production, speakers with CBD have been found to display poor maintenance of narrative theme. They also exhibit impaired global connectedness (identification of the overall point of a story) and local connectedness (connectedness between consecutive events).[18] Bob also displayed impairments in **pragmatics** and discourse. He sometimes used **pronouns** that lacked **referents** such as the use of *he* and *it* in the following utterances:

Conversation:

> he said he wouldn't let me have any (*unintelligible*) and, and then he put me in for the (1:26) to put my brain to (.) London

Cookie Theft picture description:

> she's tried to get it too

It should be noted, however, that Bob also used **pronominal reference** effectively on many other occasions as a **cohesive device**, as is illustrated by this extract from the Cookie Theft picture description task:

> a wee boy was hanging up on a (.) tis (.) is that a (.) and he's going to break his head

Bob used a further type of cohesive device – **lexical substitution** – during the Cinderella narrative task:

INV: that's the wicked stepmother, isn't it?
BOB: aye that's right
INV: um hum
BOB: it's funny they did away them you know like I never got one (.) never
INV: you never um hum
BOB: one of them (1:71)
PAR: you're lucky!

Bob appeared to draw erroneous **inferences** based on information in pictures. In the Cookie Theft picture description task, for example, Bob stated that the girl was giving cookies to the boy when, in fact, it was the boy who was giving cookies to the girl. This false statement revealed that Bob had drawn an incorrect inference about the children in the scene, an inference which compromised his understanding of their mischievous behaviour:

> the wee girl's giving him (.) the (.) cookies

As well as using incorrect information, Bob also omitted, repeated and incorrectly sequenced information in discourse. Bob's omission of information was most marked during his retelling of the Sam and Fred story. The story contains 104 words and describes a familiar scenario, the destruction caused to crops and livestock by a storm and the efforts of two farmers, Sam and Fred, to repair the damage (see Appendix). Bob recalled the events in the story as follows:

Sam and Fred (immediate recall):

> how many brothers (.) were two Frank and somebody (.) these two were doing their (*unintelligible*) (.) and then the weather come down and (.) they had to get the sh sheep out eh and the people [pʌli] came and helped them get them all into the [har] (.) that's my story

Bob's retelling of the story omitted several key points of information – the farmers had worked for several days, they were watching the weather forecasts, their crops were washed away by a large storm, the storm ripped open the door of the barn, the animals escaped from the barn, and it was nightfall before all the animals were returned to the barn. Bob did not correctly recall the names of the two brothers – one was not recalled at all and the other, Fred, was recalled incorrectly as Frank. Even in the absence of this information, and the inclusion of some incorrect information (the sheep *escaped* from the barn and were not let out by the farmers), Bob appeared to retain knowledge of narrative structure. He attempted to introduce the main protagonists. He related the main event, namely, the arrival of adverse weather conditions and some of its consequences. And he was able to describe how the farmers' problems were finally resolved. Bob's difficulties with this task were related more to memory limitations than to any lack of knowledge of the structure and function of narrative.

Bob's difficulties with the repetition and sequencing of information were most apparent during the Flowerpot Incident and the Cinderella story. The verbs *go in/ get in/got in* were used four times during Bob's telling of the Flowerpot Incident (see Appendix). Bob mentioned flowers and flowerpots five times in the same story. The final repetition of *flower* occurred long after the point at which it was relevant to the story. It resembled the **perseveration** that is known to occur in CBD:[19,20]

Flowerpot Incident:

> I think these ah (2:02) flowerpot the flowers in it and this auld boy (1:89) going to back (.) eh a flower hit him on his head and and then the flowers fell down he must have hit it with this an pulled it off and wanted to get in the door dog go in another flower dog got in and then he got in (1:57) and (1:76) ah the dog (1:60) got him up other way and he got hit, hit on the head (*laughter*) and the dog runs he away with away with the bone

Sequencing of information was impaired in Bob's narration of the Cinderella story. Bob begins his story with the final episode in the tale of Cinderella – the

Prince and Cinderella want to get married. This difficulty was compounded by the omission of a substantial amount of information and the inclusion of incorrect information – the stepmother and her daughters were 'put out' when Cinderella married the Prince:

Cinderella narrative:

> [sɪndərɛrə] an the, the (.) the, the (2:01) the (1:84) aaah her (1:81) aaah (1:71) prince (3:87) are (2:57) wanting to get married (.) and the auld mother, mother aaah (.) wild bad woman tried to stop them but her daughters (1:13) couldn't get their ugly auld feet into the, the shop [shoe] and (1:42) and the (.) when she got married (1:40) they were put out

Bob did, however, succeed in capturing the malevolent intent of the stepmother. She was described as a *wild bad woman* who tried to stop Cinderella and the Prince from getting married. This is in stark contrast to the other discourse production tasks where Bob almost consistently failed to represent the intentions and motivations of characters. During the Flowerpot Incident, Bob neglected to mention that the man was *angry* about being struck on the head by the falling flowerpot and that he entered the building with the *intention* of remonstrating with the owner of the apartment from which the pot had fallen. During the Cookie Theft picture description task, Bob stated that the sink was overflowing with water. However, he did not go on to say that this was because the mother had *forgotten* to switch off the tap as she was *daydreaming*:

Cookie Theft picture description:

> right (1:23) cookies in a box and a wee boy was hanging up on a (.) tis (.) is that a (.) and he's going to break his head and the wee girl she's tried to get it too so's as he's put them down the wee boy's on a stool and he going to get at and the wee girl's giving him (.) the (.) cookies and had her head often pushed it off properly mother's making (.) the dishes aaahhh (2:28) XXX in the dis is sis this is in (.) the water come onto the floor [*E: is there anything else you can see?*] (.) alright that's a garden yeah and there's tree out there (1:74) the hedge of another (1:53) part of the house and the curtains were pulled back away out a wee rings

Bob also failed to attribute any significance to the girl's use of gesture in the scene. The girl was gesturing to the boy to be quiet because she did not want the mother to *discover* that they were stealing cookies from the jar. Each of the italicised words used above – *angry, intention, forgotten, daydreaming, discover* – represents a cognitive or **affective mental state** that motivated the actions of the protagonists in these stories. Their omission from the narratives and other forms of discourse produced by Bob suggests that he may have problems with **theory of mind** alongside his pragmatic and discourse difficulties.[21]

COMMUNICATION PROFILE:

Speech intelligibility:

- Bob's intelligibility is reduced due to phonological and apraxic speech errors and reduced vocal volume; his conversational fluency is impaired; and he displays limited intonation and stress.

Morphology and syntax:

- Bob produces some well-formed utterances, but many utterances omit words and contain grammatical errors. Bob uses a range of inflectional morphemes (e.g. tense, number); his comprehension of syntax is functional for conversation.

Vocabulary and semantics:

- Bob makes semantic paraphasic errors; uses circumlocution; has poor semantic fluency; has word-finding difficulty in conversation. His naming of pictures is impaired but can be facilitated by use of cues. Bob makes extensive use of pauses and fillers to aid lexical retrieval; his comprehension of sentence semantics is functional for conversation.

Pragmatics:

- Bob is able to take turns in conversation; contributes utterances that are relevant and mostly informative; makes appropriate use of humour and laughter during interaction; retains understanding and use of idiomatic language; and corrects conversational misunderstanding. Sometimes Bob uses pronouns without a clear referent.

Discourse:

- Sometimes Bob draws erroneous inferences from visual information; provides inaccurate information; omits, repeats and incorrectly sequences information. He uses lexical substitution, pronominal reference and grammatical ellipsis as cohesive devices (not always accurately); he retains knowledge of narrative structure.

Cognition:

- Bob exhibits poor phonemic fluency (executive function); limited use of mental state language (theory of mind); poor planning; impulsivity; and poor immediate recall of language.

Suggestions for Further Reading

(1) Peterson, K.A., Patterson, K. and Rowe, J.B. (2019) 'Language impairment in progressive supranuclear palsy and corticobasal syndrome', *Journal of Neurology*. doi:10.1007/s00415-019-09463-1

In this article, the authors review the impact of corticobasal syndrome (and progressive supranuclear palsy) on speech and language. The overlap of CBS with PSP and other clinical conditions is addressed. The authors argue for earlier and improved language assessment in CBS.

(2) Blake, M.L., Duffy, J.R., Boeve, B.F., Ahlskog, J.E. and Maraganore, D.M. (2003) 'Speech and language disorders associated with corticobasal degeneration', *Journal of Medical Speech-Language Pathology*, 11 (3): 131–146.

The authors of this article examine speech and language characteristics in 13 individuals with autopsy-confirmed CBD. Aphasia (mostly characterised as nonfluent, or anomic) was present in over half of participants, while dysarthria and apraxia of speech were present in approximately 30% and 40% of cases, respectively. Dysarthria was mostly mixed type, with either spastic or hypokinetic features present in all affected cases.

(3) Constantinides, V.C., Paraskevas, G.P., Paraskevas, P.G., Stefanis, L. and Kapaki, E. (2019) 'Corticobasal degeneration and corticobasal syndrome: A review', *Clinical Parkinsonism & Related Disorders*, 1: 66–71.

This review examines the epidemiology, pathology, clinical features and genetics of CBD, and its most common presentation, corticobasal syndrome. CBD is a complex condition to diagnose in that clinical CBD may be caused by non-CBD pathology, while CBD pathology may present with diverse clinical phenotypes. The article describes the important role of imaging studies and biochemical markers in the diagnosis of this condition.

Questions

(1) It had taken Bob several years to obtain a medical diagnosis of his condition. His diagnosis was delayed because his neurologists were uncertain for some time about what was causing his symptoms. During conversation with the author, Bob was asked how CBD had affected his daily life. After stating that he was told he would have "two good years" and he had gone up to the "doctor's place in Coleraine", he went on to produce the following exchange with the author (INV). Examine the exchange and then answer the questions below:

BOB: and all of the young ones was, was, were here
INV: um hum
BOB: and the bigger ones the older ones was there we all other things but
INV: um hum
BOB: he said to me (.) that I'd have to come again I am (.) because (.) most of them didn't [ʌndərstɛsɪn] (understand) what was going on

(a) What type of cohesive device is Bob misapplying in this exchange?
(b) What two expressions does Bob use to achieve spatial deixis?
(c) Does Bob make appropriate use of these deictic expressions?
(d) Identify two instances where Bob uses pronominal reference in this exchange.
(e) Does Bob make appropriate use of pronominal reference?

(2) During the exchange with Bob, the author posed the following question. How would you characterise this utterance and Bob's response to it?

INV: okay so can you try telling me that story back again?
BOB: ah, ah, I'll make it short

(3) When Bob uttered "all of the young ones was, was, were here" during conversation with the author, what linguistic behaviour is he displaying? What cognitive skill must be intact for Bob to display this behaviour?

(4) Bob displayed many intact pragmatic and discourse skills. Two such skills are exemplified by the following exchange that took place during confrontation naming. Bob was shown a picture of a lobster but was unable to name it. To comprehend the author's utterance in the exchange, Bob had to understand the two features that are underlined. What are these features?

BOB: you have to put it in alive which is
INV: <u>you do</u> it's not so nice sure it's not having to do <u>that</u>
BOB: ahh it's pretty messy

The following exchange between Bob and the author occurred during the Cinderella story. Which of the two features identified previously is exemplified by the underlined words in this exchange?

INV: she drops one of her beautiful glass slippers on the steps to the palace
BOB: it was a good way to, it's good <u>she did</u>
INV: yeah it is good she left it

(5) Bob made little use of mental state language during the language tasks. However, he did use another type of language, as illustrated by the following utterances from the Cinderella narrative. What type of language is this?

> wild bad woman tried to stop them
> her daughters (1:13) couldn't get their ugly auld (old) feet into the
> the whole thing was lovely after for a while anyway

Answers

(1) Bob is misapplying lexical substitution in his use of *ones* as a substitute for *doctors*. The misapplication arises because Bob does not use *doctors* in the prior discourse context.

(a) The words *here* and *there* are used to achieve spatial deixis.

(b) Bob is presumably intending to refer to the "doctor's place in Coleraine" through use of the deictic expressions *here* and *there*. The doctor's place is at a location remote (distal) to Bob, not close (proximal) to him. So only the distal expression *there* is used correctly by Bob to refer to this location.

(c) Bob uses pronominal reference when he utters "<u>he</u> said to me" and "most of <u>them</u> didn't [ʌndərstɛsɪn] (understand)".

(d) Bob does not make appropriate use of the two instances of pronominal reference in (d) as neither pronoun has an identifiable referent in the discourse context.

(2) The author has used an indirect speech act to *request* that Bob relate the story to her. Bob's response reveals that he understands the pragmatic meaning of the author's utterance.

(3) Bob is displaying a self-initiated repair of his utterance. To undertake this repair, Bob must be able to monitor his spoken output and identify when linguistic (in this case, grammatical) errors arise.

(4) First underlined feature is *grammatical ellipsis*: "you do [have to put it in alive]". Second underlined feature is *discourse deixis*: the demonstrative pronoun *that* refers to "put it in alive".

In the second exchange between Bob and the author, Bob uses grammatical ellipsis when he says "it's good she did [drop one of her beautiful glass slippers on the steps to the palace]".

(5) Bob is using *evaluative* language in these utterances.

References

[1] Alexander, S.K., Rittman, T., Xuereb, J.H., Bak, T.H., Hodges, J.R. and Rowe, J.B. (2014) 'Validation of the new consensus criteria for the diagnosis of corticobasal degeneration', *Journal of Neurology, Neurosurgery and Psychiatry*, 85 (8): 923–927.

[2] Coyle-Gilchrist, I.T.S., Dick, K.M., Patterson, K., Vázquez Rodríquez, P., Wehmann, E., Wilcox, A., Lansdall, C.J., Dawson, K.E., Wiggins, J., Mead, S., Brayne, C. and Rowe, J.B. (2016) 'Prevalence, characteristics, and survival of frontotemporal lobar degeneration syndromes', *Neurology*, 86 (18): 1736–1743.

[3] Osaki, Y., Morita, Y., Kuwahara, T., Miyano, I. and Doi, Y. (2011) 'Prevalence of Parkinson's disease and atypical parkinsonian syndromes in a rural Japanese district', *Acta Neurologica Scandinavica*, 124 (3): 182–187.

[4] Winter, Y., Bezdolnyy, Y., Katunina, E., Avakjan, G., Reese, J.P., Klotsche, J., Oertel, W.H., Dodel, R. and Gusev, E. (2010) 'Incidence of Parkinson's disease and atypical parkinsonism: Russian population-based study', *Movement Disorders*, 25 (3): 349–356.

[5] Armstrong, M.J., Litvan, I., Lang, A.E., Bak, T.H., Bhatia, K.P., Borroni, B., Boxer, A.L., Dickson, D.W., Grossman, M., Hallett, M., Josephs, K.A., Kertesz, A., Lee, S.E., Miller, B.L., Reich, S.G., Riley, D.E., Tolosa, E., Tröster, A.I., Vidailhet, M. and Weiner, W.J. (2013) 'Criteria for the diagnosis of corticobasal degeneration', *Neurology*, 80 (5): 496–503.

[6] Dodich, A., Cerami, C., Inguscio, E., Iannaccone, S., Magnani, G., Marcone, A., Guglielmo, P., Vanoli, G., Cappa, S.F. and Perani, D. (2019) 'The clinico-metabolic correlates of language impairment in corticobasal syndrome and progressive supranuclear palsy', *NeuroImage Clinical*, 24: 102009.

[7] Frattali, C.M., Grafman, J., Patronas, N., Makhlouf, F. and Litvan, I. (2000) 'Language disturbances in corticobasal degeneration', *Neurology*, 54 (4): 990–992.

[8] Grijalvo-Perez, A.M. and Litvan, I. (2014) 'Corticobasal degeneration', *Seminars in Neurology*, 34 (2): 160–173.

[9] Lansdall, C.J., Coyle-Gilchrist, I.T.S., Jones, P.S., Vázquez Rodríguez, P., Wilcox, A., Wehmann, E., Dick, K.M., Robbins, T.W. and Rowe, J.B. (2017) 'Apathy and impulsivity in frontotemporal lobar degeneration syndromes', *Brain*, 140 (6): 1792–1807.

[10] Graham, N.L., Bak, T., Patterson, K. and Hodges, J.R. (2003) 'Language function and dysfunction in corticobasal degeneration', *Neurology*, 61 (4): 493–499.

[11] Tetzloff, K.A., Duffy, J.R., Strand, E.A., Machulda, M.M., Boland, S.M., Utianski, R.L., Botha, H., Senjem, M.L., Schwarz, C.G., Josephs, K.A. and Whitwell, J.L. (2018) 'Clinical and imaging progression over 10 years in a patient with primary progressive apraxia of speech and autopsy-confirmed corticobasal degeneration', *Neurocase*, 24 (2): 111–120.

[12] Donovan, N.J., Kendall, D.L., Moore, A.B., Rosenbek, J.C. and Gonzalez Rothi, L.J. (2007) 'Why consider impaired social language usage in a case of corticobasal degeneration', *The Clinical Neuropsychologist*, 21 (1): 190–203.

[13] Ruggeri, M., Biagioli, C., Ricci, M., Gerace, C. and Blundo, C. (2020) 'Progressive aphasia, apraxia of speech and agraphia in corticobasal degeneration: A 12-case series clinical and neuropsychological descriptive study', *International Journal of Language & Communication Disorders*, 55 (6): 867–874.

[14] Cotelli, M., Borroni, B., Manenti, R., Ginex, V., Calabria, M., Moro, A., Alberici, A., Zanetti, M., Zanetti, O., Cappa, S.F. and Padovani, A. (2007) 'Universal grammar in the frontotemporal dementia spectrum: Evidence of a selective disorder in the corticobasal degeneration syndrome', *Neuropsychologia*, 45: 3015–3023.

[15] Silveri, M.C. and Ciccarelli, N. (2007) 'The deficit for the word-class "verb" in corticobasal degeneration: Linguistic expression of the movement disorder?', *Neuropsychologia*, 45 (11): 2570–2579.

[16] Cotelli, M., Borroni, B., Manenti, R., Alberici, A., Calabria, M., Agosti, C., Arévalo, A., Ginex, V., Ortelli, P., Binetti, G., Zanetti, O., Padovani, A. and Cappa, S.F. (2006) 'Action and object naming in frontotemporal dementia, progressive supranuclear palsy, and corticobasal degeneration', *Neuropsychology*, 20 (5): 558–565.

[17] Prutting, C.A. and Kirchner, D.M. (1987) 'A clinical appraisal of the pragmatic aspects of language', *Journal of Speech and Hearing Disorders*, 52 (2): 105–119.

[18] Gross, R.G., Ash, S., McMillan, C.T., Gunawardena, D., Powers, C., Libon, D.J., Moore, P., Liang, T.-W. and Grossman, M. (2010) 'Impaired information integration contributes to communication difficulty in corticobasal syndrome', *Cognitive and Behavioral Neurology*, 23 (1): 1–7.

[19] Douglas, V.C., DeArmond, S.J., Aminoff, M.J., Miller, B.L. and Rabinovici, G.D. (2009) 'Seizures in corticobasal degeneration: A case report', *Neurocase*, 15 (4): 352–356.

[20] Mathuranath, P.S., Xuereb, J.H., Bak, T. and Hodges, J.R. (2000) 'Corticobasal ganglionic degeneration and/or frontotemporal dementia? A report of two overlap cases and review of literature', *Journal of Neurology, Neurosurgery and Psychiatry*, 68 (3): 304–312.

[21] Poletti, M. and Bonuccelli, U. (2012) 'Impairment of affective theory of mind in corticobasal degeneration', *Journal of Neuropsychiatry and the Clinical Neurosciences*, 24 (1): E7. doi:10.1176/appi.neuropsych.11010021.

CASE STUDY 2

Progressive Supranuclear Palsy

KEY FACTS AND FIGURES:

- Progressive supranuclear palsy (PSP) is a tauopathy that is characterized clinically by progressive supranuclear ophthalmoparesis, bradykinesia, and axial rigidity, amongst other symptoms. Phenotypic heterogeneity in PSP is associated with variability of regional distribution and severity of abnormal tau accumulation and neuronal loss.[1]
- The incidence of PSP is approximately 1 per 100,000 and the prevalence is approximately 5 per 100,000.[2] These figures can vary with geographical region. For example, the prevalence of PSP is estimated to be 6.4 per 100,000 in London, UK and 17.90 per 100,000 in Yonago, Japan.[3,4] The mean age of onset is 63 years and median survival is 7 years.[5]
- A wide range of symptoms can occur in PSP. In one clinical sample, motor symptoms (100%) were most common at baseline, followed by cognitive (e.g. memory) and behavioural (e.g. obsessive-compulsive behaviours) symptoms (89%), systemic (e.g. incontinence) and bulbar (e.g. dysphagia) symptoms (80%), and sleep disturbances (60%). Early dysphagia and early cognitive symptoms are unfavourable predictors of survival in PSP.[6,7]
- The major genetic risk factor for sporadic PSP is a common variant in the gene encoding microtubule-associated protein tau (MAPT). There is also evidence that PSP is associated with environmental risk factors (e.g. drinking well water).[8,9]

DOI: 10.4324/9781003153559-3

- Speech and language are impaired in PSP. In one clinical sample of 17 individuals with PSP, apraxia of speech (AoS) was identified in 76.47% of the sample. Impairments were also identified in semantic fluency (58.8%), naming (52.9%), sentence comprehension (52.9%), sentence repetition (23.5%), reading (41.2%) and semantic association (7%). Orthographic errors occurred in 28.6% of the sample.[10]
- Aphasia of similar severity to that seen in progressive non-fluent aphasia (PNFA) is reported in PSP.[11] Atypical PSP, in which there is a shift in pathology from subcortical grey and brainstem regions to neocortical regions, can present as AoS and PNFA.[12]

Background

Harry (not his real name) is 72;7 years old. He is a retired computer manager. He is married and has a daughter and two granddaughters, aged 8 and 10 years. Harry's daughter lives in a city in Hertfordshire, England. Harry and his wife make regular trips to visit her and her two children. Harry was diagnosed with PSP in July 2016. However, his wife and other family members noticed signs that all was not well as far back as 1995. There were changes in his posture and length of stride. There was a loss of facial expression and withdrawal from social activities. However, Harry's wife acknowledges that it is difficult to know which, if any, of these changes in motor skills, personality and interests were due to PSP or were related to other factors. Harry and his wife are keen to participate in research into PSP, and both have agreed to donate their brains to medical research.

Harry has had a complicated diagnostic history. He was initially diagnosed by a neurologist in 2006 with **Parkinson's disease**. In 2015, Harry was admitted to hospital after a serious fall. He was under the care of a different neurologist. PSP was suspected at this stage and was subsequently diagnosed in 2016. Harry's father died at 68 years of age with early-onset **Alzheimer's disease** (AD) and his paternal grandmother spent 20 years in a hospital in Belfast unable to care for herself. Given that tau proteins are found in both PSP and AD, Harry's new neurologist had blood samples taken to perform genetic testing. Currently, he is seeing a neurologist approximately every 6 months. Recently, Harry's health has been compromised by infections related to a permanent catheter. This is used to treat an enlarged prostate gland that was diagnosed in 2015. Between November 2017 and April 2018, Harry had seven infections that caused confusion and exacerbated his PSP symptoms.

Clinical Symptoms

Harry's wife reports significant movement problems. He has a rigid gait and "odd" movement of his feet. The left side of his body "would lead you to suspect a **stroke** down his left side". Although Harry can walk for long distances, the length of his stride has become short. His balance has been badly affected and he falls every day. Falls are most common when he gets up from chairs, walks backwards or changes direction. In March 2018, Harry had a bone density scan to see if he required calcium to strengthen his bones to cope with his regular falls. His wife reports that his rugby training has taught him how to fall properly and that hospital staff commented on how well he fell when he was in hospital. Harry uses a wheelchair in situations where he could fall and injure others. Tasks that involve movement other than walking are also difficult for him to perform. Harry has received physiotherapy. Occupational therapy has arranged for a through-the-floor lift to be installed at home.

Harry exhibits significant oculomotor and visual difficulties. His pupils are "pinpoint" (reduced pupil diameter). His eyes do not move up and down at all (vertical gaze palsy) and move from side to side very little (horizontal gaze palsy). This causes double vision (**diplopia**). He is seen by an ophthalmologist regularly and has glasses with prisms to prevent double vision. Prior to his diagnosis, Harry sat tests for Mensa at Queen's University Belfast and became a member in 2002. However, he now displays some cognitive difficulties. He experiences **short-term memory** loss. He can also display intermittent confusion, particularly when he is awakening from sleep. His wife finds it difficult to convince him that what he is saying is not true. For example, he may search for something that he never had. There are also marked personality changes. Harry was head boy at school, captain of 1st fifteen in rugby and a scout leader for 30 years. His wife reports that the personality traits that he now exhibits are not those expected of someone in these positions.

Harry has experienced several other symptoms. His wife reports excessive salivation, a feature related to reduced swallowing in PSP.[13] Harry's nose runs more than normal, and he is often unaware that this is happening. He has also experienced a loss of the sense of smell. While marked olfactory dysfunction is a feature of Parkinson's disease, it is generally not found in PSP.[14] Harry's wife reports a reduction in his use of facial expression. As a result, people assume that he is not aware of what is going on and that he is suffering from **dementia**. His wife describes some impairment of his emotional responses to situations, a behaviour that she attributes to his reduced use of facial expression. For example, she states that he displays a lack of embarrassment and annoyance when he falls, even though those around him are shocked and concerned. People often comment that Harry is fond of his food due to the speed at which he eats. He also crams food into his mouth, a behaviour associated with **impulsivity** in PSP.[15] Because of food cramming and poor manual dexterity, food goes onto his clothes and the floor.

Daily Activities

PSP has had a negative impact on all of Harry's daily activities. He has had to stop driving, playing golf and football, cooking and working in the garden. He is not able to perform general household tasks. Harry can play bowls. Due to his visual problems and difficulties with manual dexterity, he cannot undertake activities that require the use of a keyboard. He is unable to go out on his own because of the risk of falls. This has led to a loss of independence.

Medication

Harry takes a range of medications, only some of which are related to management of PSP. To treat his **hypertension**, he takes Lisinopril 2.5 mg tablets (one daily in the morning). For treatment of his enlarged prostate, he takes Finasteride 5 mg tablets (one daily). Harry also takes Sinemet Plus tablets (one three times a day, morning, noon and night), half Sinemet CR 125 mg tablets (one at night) and Sinemet 12.5/50 mg tablets (one three times a day, morning, noon and night). Sinemet® is a combination of carbidopa and **levodopa** for the treatment of Parkinson's disease and syndrome. Finally, Harry also takes Gatalin XL 16 mg prolonged release capsules (one daily). Gatalin XL is indicated for the symptomatic treatment of mild to moderately severe dementia of the Alzheimer type.

Communication

Harry's wife reports several communication difficulties. She describes how he finds words "hard to get out" and that he has "a sort of stutter". When words do come out, they are heard as a mumble and he must then repeat himself. Harry speaks with low volume. His wife reports that he interprets utterances literally. She recounted an episode where Harry was being tested. He was asked to produce words that begin with the letter 'T'. One of the words he produced was *TomTom* (a brand of satnav). When his wife later asked him why he did not just say *Tom*, he responded that he was asked to name *things*. When Harry is in the company of others, he can follow conversation but cannot think of what to say to join in. Harry says that he has never been a conversationalist. He has attended speech and language therapy several times and has been given speech exercises which he tries to remember to do regularly. The therapist is "happy" with his speech and is "keeping a close watch" on his swallowing. Harry and his wife have no plans for another speech therapy appointment, but they know that they can get one if they think it is necessary. Harry attends the Parkinson's choir every Saturday where he participates in a programme of exercises and songs that are designed to help speech. Harry's speed of reading has slowed down, which his wife attributes to his eye problems.

The author visited Harry and his wife at home in the afternoon of 25 July 2018. An audio-recording was made in the dining room of their house as Harry undertook several language tasks. The recording was stopped at the halfway stage for a tea break. Harry was attentive and focused throughout the session. He was responsive to all questions and cooperative during the tasks. He did not initiate communication. This was in part explained by the fact that most activities required him to respond to questions and instructions from the author. Additionally, however, it was clear from the outset of the interaction that Harry's wife directed conversation by asking him questions to which she already knew the answers (e.g. *What happens when we are out with people?*), by instructing him to talk about certain things (e.g. *Tell Louise about the library at Queens*) and by providing him with the first letter and sound of words that he was struggling to produce (e.g. *Begins with an 'R'*). She also explicitly corrected what he said on several occasions (e.g. *No, you went to Queens first*). This style of conversation had restricted Harry to the role of a passive respondent and was probably a more exaggerated form of their premorbid pattern of communication.

Dysarthria in individuals with PSP has prominent hypokinetic and spastic components with less prominent ataxic components.[16] Although Harry spoke with low volume, his production of speech sounds was largely intact. There were few instances of unintelligibility during the test session with the author (INV). When speech production difficulties did arise, Harry produced one or two syllables of the target word and then appeared to run out of breath support for the rest of the word. Occasionally, his wife (PAR) reminded him to take a deep breath:

HAR: I was a computer manager there for (.)
INV: un hum
HAR: a num (.) hee (2:20)
PAR: deep breath
INV: um hum
HAR: number of years

Low volume and loudness decay related to poor breath support for speech are features of **hypokinetic dysarthria** in PSP.[16] The repetition of sounds, words and phrases is also a feature of speech production in PSP.[16] Extensive function word repetition is reported in a French-speaking adult with PSP.[17] On a few occasions, Harry repeated the initial sounds and syllables of words in the lead-up to producing a word:

[puːtɛrz] (computers) suh, suh, sys, system, system in their library (.) li, li, library

This compromised his conversational **fluency**. But so too did the use of lengthy timed pauses, which appeared to be related to sentence **planning** and **lexical retrieval** problems:

they em (2:62) they (6:76) the door of the barn was blown off

That Harry may have needed increased time in which to plan his utterances is also suggested by his poor performance on **phonemic fluency**, a test of **executive function** and lexical retrieval. Harry produced only two words beginning with the letter 'F' in 60 seconds. This figure is consistent with reports of poor phonemic fluency scores in PSP in the literature. On letter/phonemic fluency tasks, up to 50% of people with PSP have been found to name fewer than three words per minute, 80% fewer than five words, and 85% fewer than nine words.[18] A cut-off score of seven words or less beginning with the letter 'F' has been found to support a diagnosis of PSP.[19]

Harry displayed intact knowledge of the morphological structure of words, with a range of inflectional and derivational morphemes used correctly during the test session:

education board<u>s</u> (*-s plural number*)

I was do<u>ing</u> (*-ing progressive aspect*)

join<u>ed</u> the boat (*-ed past tense*)

the men<u>'s</u> choir (*-'s genitive*)

it was sharpen<u>ed</u> (*-ed passive participle*)

lived happi<u>ly</u> ever after (*-ly derivational suffix*)

very enjoy<u>able</u> (*-able derivational suffix*)

Harry was able to use complex **syntax**. During the sentence generation task, Harry produced the following sentence that contained the target words *chair, doctor* and *sit*:

> the patient was shown into the doctor's surgery (.) where he was asked to sit on a chair

This sentence contains two **passive voice** constructions (e.g. *he was asked*), an **infinitive clause** (*to sit on a chair*), and an adverbial **subordinate clause** (*where he was asked to sit on a chair*). Harry used equally complex grammatical structures during conversation and **discourse** production tasks:

Conversation:

> I was managing a computer system <u>that was being run by the five boards</u>
>
> (*passive relative clause*)

Flowerpot Incident:

> man was walking along the road with his dog <u>when a flowerpot fell off a balcony and hit him in the head</u>
>
> (*adverbial subordinate clause*)

Harry's receptive syntax was also an area of relative strength. He was able to comprehend utterances with embedded clauses and other complex structures during the test session:

> you also said <u>that you're not a big conversationalist</u>
>
> *(declarative subordinate clause)*

> can you just tell me everything <u>that you see</u> going on in this picture?
>
> *(relative clause)*

Harry's lexical-semantic abilities displayed a more uneven pattern of performance. Harry exhibited excellent lexical retrieval during **confrontation naming**, obtaining a score of 100% on this language task. This result is consistent with reports of intact or almost intact confrontation naming in PSP.[20] However, this performance was not carried over into spontaneous conversation, where Harry displayed evidence of word-finding difficulties. Harry's wife used phonemic (sound), orthographic (letter), and lexical cues to trigger production of target words. Only the latter type of cue achieved naming of the target word:

Lexical cue:

HAR: after the civil service I went to (.) to (2:03) em (.)
PAR: Ulster …
HAR: Ulsterbus
INV: oh, okay, right, right

Phonemic cue:

HAR: was a (.) river cruise on the Danube (.) we went (.) initially to (.) am (2:00)
PAR: ma, ma, Germany, Munich
HAR: Munich
INV: um hum

Orthographic cue:

PAR: what did I look up last night?
HAR: oh yes, another *(unintelligible)* river cruise
INV: *(laughter)* another
HAR: cruise
PAR: where?
HAR: am (2:71)
PAR: begins with an 'R'
HAR: (3:35)
PAR: The Rhine
HAR: what?

PAR: The Rhine
HAR: The Rhine yes

Notwithstanding these word-finding difficulties, Harry did not use **circumlo-cutions** or produce semantic paraphasic errors. There were also no visual errors in his naming. This is contrary to reports of visual errors in naming in PSP,[21] where such errors are attributed to gaze palsy and other visual difficulties that are common in PSP.[20] Harry also did not appear to have difficulty in the naming and comprehension of action verbs, both of which are reported to be impaired in PSP.[22,23]

Harry's superior confrontation naming over letter (phonemic) fluency sug-gests that his marked fluency deficit may be related more to problems of **execu-tive function** than to any impairment of language as such. This is confirmed by Harry's better performance on semantic (category) fluency than **letter fluency**. Harry obtained a **semantic fluency** score of 9 animal names in 60 seconds. This is consistent with the finding in PSP of severe impairment of letter fluency and more moderate deficits in **category fluency**.[20]

Harry's other semantic skills were an area of strength. He was able to use a range of **semantic roles** to represent different participants including agent (e.g. _The man_ kissed her hand), patient (e.g. _The water_ was spilling out of the sink), and instrument (e.g. The door of the barn was blown off by _the storm_). Harry used verbs that revealed an ability to express semantic distinctions in different action processes. For example, the verb _comment_ in the following utterance captures an action that takes place over time (is 'durative') but has no inherent endpoint (is 'unbounded'):

look what they were doing and things and _comment_ on it

The use of _joined_ in the utterance below also captures an action that is spread over time. But unlike _comment_, it has an inherent endpoint and expresses a 'bounded' action:

and _joined_ the boat there (2:25) and just cruised

Harry displayed strengths and weaknesses in **pragmatics** and **discourse** during the test session. He was aware of the expectation to be maximally informative in conversation. This is clearly illustrated by the following exchange. Harry's use of "five boards" did not allow the author to determine the type of boards Harry was talking about, a pragmatic shortcoming for which he felt the need to apologise:

HAR: I was managing a computer system that was being run by the five boards
INV: okay
HAR: em (.) it was interesting

INV: yes, is this the health boards?
HAR: no, it's the education boards
INV: education boards
HAR: sorry

The expectation to be informative led Harry to produce a complete description of the actions of the woman and the two children in the Cookie Theft picture, and the gentleman and his dog in the Flowerpot Incident:

Cookie Theft picture description:

> the lady of the house is doing the dishes and the water was spilling out of the sink onto the floor (2:01) at her feet, the children were (2:18) trying to steal cookies (.) from the cookie jar (.) and the boy was standing on a stool and was falling off it (.) and the girl was just trying to take the cookies from him (3:71) that's basically it.

Flowerpot Incident:

> right (.) man was walking along the road with his dog when a flowerpot fell off a balcony and hit him in the head, he was very cross about this and ranted and raved at the (.) the balcony (.) then he went into the house that it was (.) part of (.) and rapped on the door, when the woman came out she saw the dog with him and was very kind to it and gave it a bone so the man (2:75) kissed her hand and said thank you very much (.) then dog left

Through their use of visual information in pictures, these discourse production tasks placed reduced demands on Harry's **working memory**. In the absence of this visual support, however, Harry omitted significant amounts of information during discourse production. This was evident during Cinderella narration. Harry omitted several important events, including the king's decision to invite all eligible women to a ball at the palace, the receipt of an invitation to the ball by Cinderella's stepmother and the use of a magic spell by the fairy godmother. The omission of this information, and other information, left listeners with the impression that Harry had 'skipped over' complete episodes in the story, indicated by **[XXX]** below:

Cinderella narration:

> Cinderella was (2:20) ah (.) the daughter of a house (.) that their mother had died and she had a wicked stepmother take over (.) and her two (.) ugly sisters as well (2:69) ah am ah (13:58) Cinderella had to do all the

dishes an things in the house (.) and was kept more as a skivvy rather than as a (3:25) a ah as (.) su, su, su, su, su, sister (2:71) **[XXX]** and then em (2:96) she met the there was a fairy godmother arrived in the house (.) and (.) dressed her up for the (.) visit to the ball where the prince was (.) and (4:70) she (3:00) went to the ball with her ugly sisters who were (.) cast out to one side (.) and she went (.) um (.) **[XXX]** when the su, clock struck twelve she had to run (.) to get home before she cha, cha, changed back into her own clothes (.) and she dropped her slipper (.) and the prince (3:67) wanted to meet this girl again (.) so he took the slipper and went round the countryside (.) until he found (2:00) someone it fitted (2:17) when he went to Cinderella's house the, the sisters fought over who (.) who, who (2:05) who, who would fit (2:18) but em (.) Cinderella (2:67) eventually (2:76) got back with the prince and lived happily ever after.

Harry also struggled to fulfil other discourse expectations. During immediate recall of the Sam and Fred story, Harry succeeded in capturing the main events in the story. So, he produced *informative* discourse. However, the events in the story were related in the wrong order. Two key events – the storm blew the door off the barn and the animals escaped – are mentioned *after* the arrival of local people to assist the two farmers when, in fact, these events preceded the villagers' arrival:

Sam and Fred (immediate recall):

Fred and Sam were brothers who farmed (.) am they, they were looking at the weather wondering when it was going to change (.) em (.) but they kept working and (.) having spent two days working (.) the weather suddenly changed (.) and the rain came down very heavily (2:16) they um (2:62) started to clear up their mess and then (.) the people from the town came out to help them (.) as well they em (2:62) they (6:76) the door of the barn was blown off by the storm and the animals escaped and they managed to get their animals back in together again but it took most of the day

Aside from information management, Harry displayed a range of other pragmatic and discourse skills. He was able to use and understand **cohesive devices** across different discourse contexts. In the following conversational exchange with the author, Harry used *ones* as a substitute for *cruises*. Additionally, he understood the author when she used *third* <u>one</u> as a substitute for *third* <u>cruise</u>:

INV: so, would cruises be something that you would do quite often?
HAR: no, this is probably our third cruise
INV: a third <u>one</u>
HAR: the other <u>ones</u> were river or sea cruises, sea cruises

Pronominal reference was also skilfully used by Harry to achieve **cohesion** with other utterances. In the exchange below, Harry used the **demonstrative pronoun** *that* to refer to the playing of bowls in his preceding conversational utterance:

HAR: I play bowls
INV: you play bowls good um hum
HAR: <u>that</u>'s about the only
PAR: what about Saturday afternoons?
HAR: pardon, oh yes, the Parkinson's choir as well

In the utterance below, the demonstrative pronoun *that* is used to refer to the establishment of a computer system in a school in Scotland, an activity that was described by Harry across several earlier conversational turns:

> <u>that</u> was just a weekend thing that we went to

Harry also used grammatical **ellipsis** to achieve cohesion in conversation, as the italicised extract in the following example illustrates:

INV: so that's made a positive impression on you
HAR: it has [*made a positive impression on me*] yes

Harry made accurate use of **deixis** during the test session. This included *spatial deixis* during conversation about his river cruise in Germany. Harry used the **adverb** *there* to refer to the German town Passau:

PAR: went from Munich to Passau
HAR: Passau
INV: okay
HAR: and joined the boat <u>there</u> (2:25) and just cruised

During conversation about his work history, Harry used *temporal deixis*. The adjective *last* was used to refer to the 18-month period immediately prior to the author's conversation with Harry:

INV: how long did you do this work, was this your full career?
HAR: no, no, this was just for the <u>last</u> about 18 months

Harry used several expressions that contained **presuppositions**. In the utterance below, the verb *managed* presupposes that the two farmers *tried* to return their escaped animals to the barn. This presupposition is appropriate in the context of the Sam and Fred story:

> they <u>managed</u> to get their animals back in

However, the iterative expression *again* in the following utterance presupposes that the prince had met Cinderella *before*. But an examination of Harry's Cinderella narrative shows that all we are told is that Cinderella visited the ball and that the prince was there, not that the prince met Cinderella. Of course, we can *infer* that this meeting occurred. But it is arguable whether Harry has undertaken the pragmatic work that is required to make his use of presupposition appropriate on this occasion:

> and the prince (3:67) wanted to meet this girl <u>again</u>

Conversational repair is a complex pragmatic language skill. Harry was able to participate in repair sequences during conversation. In the following exchange with his wife (PAR), he undertakes other-initiated self-repair during talk about his interests and hobbies:

HAR: oh, I'm in the church choir
PAR: not the church choir
HAR: the church choir but the men's choir in the church

Finally, Harry used only three mental state terms during the discourse production tasks. These terms captured cognitive and **affective mental states**:

> they were looking at the weather, <u>wondering</u> when it was going to change
> the prince (3:67) <u>wanted</u> to meet this girl again
> he was very <u>cross</u> about this

The low frequency of these terms and the complete omission of mental state language like *forgetting* and *daydreaming* from the Cookie Theft picture description task are consistent with reports of cognitive and affective ToM deficits in PSP.[24,25]

COMMUNICATION PROFILE:

Speech intelligibility:

- Harry speaks with low volume and poor timing of breathing for speech results in loss of air in the middle of words; articulation of speech sounds is intact for the most part; conversational fluency is sometimes compromised by multiple repetitions of the first syllable of words and use of lengthy pauses; Harry has limited intonation and stress.

Morphology and syntax:

- Harry's use of inflectional and derivational morphology is intact; he is able to use and understand complex syntax across different discourse contexts.

Vocabulary and semantics:

- Harry's naming of objects during confrontation naming is intact; Harry experiences word-finding difficulty in conversation; the use of cues to prompt target words is minimally effective; Harry is able to use various semantic roles to represent participants in a situation; he uses verbs that represent different semantic distinctions in action processes; Harry's semantic fluency is moderately impaired.

Pragmatics:

- Harry is able to take turns in conversation and contribute relevant, informative utterances; he does not initiate conversation, use laughter or engage in humour; facial expression and gesture are lacking. Harry tends to interpret language literally. Harry uses deixis and presupposition; participates in conversational repair; and he is aware of the need to fulfil conversational expectations relating to the informativeness of an utterance.

Discourse:

- Harry omits information in discourse when there is no pictorial support. He occasionally reports events in the wrong order in narratives. He can use and understand cohesive devices including lexical substitution, pronominal reference and ellipsis.

Cognition:

- Harry displays reduced use of mental state language (theory of mind); very poor phonemic fluency (executive function); some impulsivity; and reduced emotional expression. His memory contributes to reduced information during discourse production.

Suggestions for Further Reading

(1) Kim, J.-H. and McCann, C.M. (2015) 'Communication impairments in people with progressive supranuclear palsy: A tutorial', *Journal of Communication Disorders*, 56: 76–87.

This tutorial examines clinical and neuropathological features of PSP and reviews the findings of published studies of communication in the disorder. Motor speech production and expressive and receptive language are addressed, as well as cognitive (executive function) deficits in PSP. The

assessment and treatment of clients with PSP by speech-language pathologists are also considered.

(2) Strand, E.A. (2010) 'Corticobasal ganglionic degeneration and progressive
supranuclear palsy: Clinical and speech-language characteristics', *Perspectives
on Neurophysiology and Neurogenic Speech and Language Disorders*, 20 (2): 45–49.

This article describes the neuroanatomical correlates, pathophysiology,
and clinical presentation of PSP. Strand also examines speech and language
disorders associated with PSP, including dysarthria, progressive nonfluent
aphasia, and progressive apraxia of speech.

(3) Golbe, L.I. (2014) 'Progressive supranuclear palsy', *Seminars in Neurology*, 34
(2): 151–159.

This article provides an accessible overview of the epidemiology, genetics,
clinical features, diagnosis, prognosis, and treatment of PSP. It is an excellent
medical primer on this disorder for speech-language pathologists with little
or no prior knowledge of PSP.

Questions

(1) Like other neurodegenerative dyads, Harry and his wife displayed a pattern of interaction that was governed by several conversational moves. These
moves were initiated by Harry's wife. They restricted Harry to the role of
a passive conversational partner who merely responded to his wife's verbal
prompts. They included the use of (i) direct questions; (ii) explicit commands; (iii) sound and syllable cues; (iv) letter cues; (v) sentence completion
prompts; and (vi) explicit corrections. The following utterances were produced by Harry's wife during the test session. Assign each of them to one of
the above categories:

   (a) *List the other places you went*
   (b) *From there you went to …*
   (c) *What countries did we pass through?*
   (d) *What did I do last night?*
   (e) *Not the church choir*
   (f) *You just …*

(2) Harry was able to use and understand pragmatic and discourse features of
language. Several utterances from Harry's exchange with the author (INV)
and his wife (PAR) are shown below. Identify the pragmatic and discourse
behaviour exemplified by the utterances in (a) to (e):

   (a) **HAR:** there was a computer system (.) it was running the University of
   Ulster
   (b) **INV:** can you tell me a bit about that?
   HAR: was a (.) river cruise

(c) **HAR:** I went to (.) to (2:03) em (.) Ulsterbus I was a computer manager <u>there</u> for (.)

(d) **HAR:** we went to a school in Scotland to see (.) to see if we could (.) introduce […] system in their library
PAR: the <u>one</u> Princess Anne went to

(e) **HAR:** man was walking along the road with <u>his</u> dog when a flowerpot fell off a balcony and hit <u>him</u> in the head

(3) Harry's wife posed several direct questions to him during the test session. Some of these questions are shown below. What pragmatic feature of these questions sets them apart from most other questions used in conversation?

> *What happens when we are out with people?*
> *What countries did we pass through?*
> *What did I look up last night?*

(4) Harry produced the following utterances during the test session. What do these utterances have in common? What do they reveal about Harry's language skills?

> that was just a weekend thing that we went to
> look what they were doing and things
> trees are special things
> Cinderella had to do all the dishes an things in the house
> they started to get their animals in (.) and things
> got them all into their (.) barns and things

(5) Examine the exchange below between Harry (HAR), the author (INV) and Harry's wife (PAR). What is the author planning to do at T3? What happens to these plans between T4 and T8? Does the author return to her plan at T3 at a later point in the exchange?

T1 INV: okay so you you've actually worked in quite a number of different sorts of sectors
T2 HAR: yes, ah ha
T3 INV: you've worked in
T4 PAR: Queen's
T5 INV: ah ha
T6 PAR: University of Ulster
T7 INV: right
T8 PAR: and he
T9 INV: so, so you've been at universities, you've been at the Education Board, you've been in private companies like Ulsterbus
T10 HAR: um hum

Answers

(1) (a) explicit command
   (b) sentence completion prompt
   (c) direct question
   (d) direct question
   (e) explicit correction
   (f) sentence completion prompt

(2) (a) anaphoric reference (cohesive device): pronoun *it* refers to the preceding noun phrase *a computer system*
   (b) indirect speech act (a request)
   (c) anaphoric *there*: adverb *there* refers to *Ulsterbus*
   (d) lexical substitution (cohesive device): use of *one* as a substitute for *school*
   (e) anaphoric reference (cohesive device): use of *his* and *him* to refer to preceding noun phrase *man*

(3) Normally, when speakers pose questions in conversation, they do not know the answers to these questions. This lack of knowledge is a pragmatic condition on the felicitous use of questions. However, when Harry's wife asks him questions, she does so with knowledge of their answers in mind. These questions are pragmatically anomalous and have the status of 'test' questions – they are intended to test Harry and are not genuinely information-seeking questions.

(4) These utterances all use the non-specific lexeme *thing(s)*. The use of this word suggests a word-finding difficulty on Harry's part, with *thing(s)* serving as a substitute for other words that Harry is unable to retrieve.

(5) At T3, the author is planning to summarise the different jobs that Harry has undertaken as part of his work history. The author abandons these plans between T4 and T8, as Harry's wife dominates the exchange by listing his different jobs. Finally, at T9 the author succeeds in providing Harry with this summary which he then confirms at T10.

References

[1] Ling, H. (2016) 'Clinical approach to progressive supranuclear palsy', *Journal of Movement Disorders*, 9 (1): 3–13.
[2] Golbe, L.I. (2008) 'The epidemiology of progressive supranuclear palsy', in C. Duyckaerts and I. Litvan (eds), *Handbook of Clinical Neurology, Volume 89: Dementias*, Edinburgh: Elsevier, 457–459.
[3] Schrag, A., Ben-Shlomo, Y. and Quinn, N.P. (1999) 'Prevalence of progressive supranuclear palsy and multiple system atrophy: A cross-sectional study', *Lancet*, 354 (9192): 1771–1775.
[4] Takigawa, H., Kitayama, M., Wada-Isoe, K., Kowa, H. and Nakashima, K. (2016) 'Prevalence of progressive supranuclear palsy in Yonago: Change throughout a decade', *Brain and Behavior*, 6 (12): e00557. doi:10.1002/brb3.557
[5] Golbe, L.I. (2014) 'Progressive supranuclear palsy', *Seminars in Neurology*, 34 (2): 151–159.

[6] Arena, J.E., Weigand, S.D., Whitwell, J.L., Hassan, A., Eggers, S.D., Litvan, G.U. and Josephs, K.A. (2016) 'Progressive supranuclear palsy: Progression and survival', *Journal of Neurology*, 263 (2): 380–389.

[7] Glasmacher, S.A., Leigh, P.N. and Saha, R.A. (2017) 'Predictors of survival in progressive supranuclear palsy and multiple system atrophy: A systematic review and meta-analysis', *Journal of Neurology, Neurosurgery, and Psychiatry*, 88 (5): 402–411.

[8] Dickson, D.W., Rademakers, R. and Hutton, M.L. (2007) 'Progressive supranuclear palsy: Pathology and genetics', *Brain Pathology*, 17 (1): 74–82.

[9] Litvan, I., Lees, P.S., Cunningham, C.R., Rai, S.N., Cambon, A.C., Standaert, D.G., Marras, C., Juncos, J., Riley, D., Reich, S., Hall, D., Kluger, B., Bordelon, Y., Shprecher, D.R. for ENGENE-PSP (2016) 'Environmental and occupational risk factors for progressive supranuclear palsy: Case-control study', *Movement Disorders*, 31 (5): 644–652.

[10] Catricalà, E., Boschi, V., Cuoco, S., Galiano, F., Picillo, M., Gobbi, E., Miozzo, A., Chesi, C., Esposito, V., Santangelo, G., Pellecchia, M.T., Borsa, V.M., Barone, P., Garrard, P., Iannaccone, S. and Cappa, S.F. (2019) 'The language profile of progressive supranuclear palsy', *Cortex*, 115: 294–308.

[11] Burrell, J.R., Ballard, K.J., Halliday, G.M. and Hodges, J.R. (2018) 'Aphasia in progressive supranuclear palsy: As severe as progressive non-fluent aphasia', *Journal of Alzheimer's Disease*, 61 (2): 705–715.

[12] Josephs, K.A., Boeve, B.F., Duffy, J.R., Smith, G.E., Knopman, D.S., Parisi, J.E., Petersen, R.C. and Dickson, D.W. (2005) 'Atypical progressive supranuclear palsy underlying progressive apraxia of speech and nonfluent aphasia', *Neurocase*, 11 (4): 283–296.

[13] Johnston, B.T., Castell, J.A., Stumacher, S., Colcher, A., Gideon, R.M., Li, Q. and Castell, D.O. (1997) 'Comparison of swallowing function in Parkinson's disease and progressive supranuclear palsy', *Movement Disorders*, 12 (3): 322–327.

[14] Katzenschlager, R. and Lees, A.J. (2004) 'Olfaction and Parkinson's syndrome: Its role in differential diagnosis', *Current Opinion in Neurology*, 17 (4): 417–423.

[15] Rittman, T., Coyle-Gilchrist, I.T.S. and Rowe, J.B. (2016) 'Managing cognition in progressive supranuclear palsy', *Neurodegenerative Disease Management*, 6 (6): 499–508.

[16] Kluin, K., Gilman, S., Foster, N., Sima, A., D'Amato, C., Bruch, L., Bluemlein, L., Little, R. and Johanns, L. (2001) 'Neuropathological correlates of dysarthria in progressive supranuclear palsy', *Archives of Neurology*, 58 (2): 265–269.

[17] Lebrun, Y., Devreux, F. and Rousseau, J.-J. (1986) 'Language and speech in a patient with a clinical diagnosis of progressive supranuclear palsy', *Brain and Language*, 27 (2): 247–256.

[18] Gerstenecker, A. (2017) 'The neuropsychology (broadly conceived) of multiple system atrophy, progressive supranuclear palsy, and corticobasal degeneration', *Archives of Clinical Neuropsychology*, 32 (7): 861–875.

[19] Fiorenzato, E., Weis, L., Falup-Pecurariu, C., Diaconu, S., Siri, C., Reali, E., Pezzoli, G., Bisiacchi, P., Antonini, A. and Biundo, R. (2016) 'Montreal Cognitive Assessment (MoCA) and Mini-Mental State Examination (MMSE) performance in progressive supranuclear palsy and multiple system atrophy', *Journal of Neural Transmission*, 123 (12): 1435–1442.

[20] Peterson, K.A., Patterson, K. and Rowe, J.B. (2019) 'Language impairment in progressive supranuclear palsy and corticobasal syndrome', *Journal of Neurology*, 268 (3): 796–809.

[21] Podoll, K., Schwarz, M. and Noth, J. (1991) 'Language functions in progressive supranuclear palsy', *Brain*, 114 (3): 1457–1472.

[22] Daniele, A., Barbier, A., Di Giuda, D., Vita, M.G., Piccininni, C., Spinelli, P., Tondo, G., Fasano, A., Colosimo, C., Giordano, A. and Gainotti, G. (2013) 'Selective impairment of action-verb naming and comprehension in progressive supranuclear palsy', *Cortex*, 49 (4): 948–960.

[23] Cotelli, M., Borroni, B., Manenti, R., Alberici, A., Calabria, M., Agosti, C., Arévalo, A., Ginex, V., Ortelli, P., Binetti, G., Zanetti, O., Padovani, A. and Cappa, S.F. (2006) 'Action and object naming in frontotemporal dementia, progressive supranuclear palsy, and corticobasal degeneration', *Neuropsychology*, 20 (5): 558–565.

[24] Ghosh, B.C., Calder, A.J., Peers, P.V., Lawrence, A.D., Acosta-Cabronero, J., Pereira, J.M., Hodges, J.R. and Rowe, J.B. (2012) 'Social cognitive deficits and their neural correlates in progressive supranuclear palsy', *Brain*, 135 (7): 2089–2102.

[25] Shany-Ur, T., Poorzand, P., Grossman, S., Growdon, M., Jang, J., Ketelle, R., Miller, B.L. and Rankin, K.P. (2012) 'Comprehension of insincere communication in neurodegenerative disease: Lies, sarcasm, and theory of mind', *Cortex*, 48 (10): 1329–1341.

CASE STUDY 3

Huntington's Disease

KEY FACTS AND FIGURES:

- Huntington's disease (HD) is a neurodegenerative disease that is caused by a dominantly inherited CAG (cytosine, adenine, guanine) trinucleotide repeat expansion in the huntingtin gene on chromosome 4.[1]
- HD has an incidence of 0.38 per 100,000 per year. The worldwide prevalence of HD is 2.71 per 100,000. The prevalence of HD is higher in Europe, North America and Australia (5.70 per 100,000) than in Asia (0.40 per 100,000).[2]
- The average age of HD onset is between 40 and 50 years. Some 25% of patients experience their initial symptoms after 50 years of age. Onset before the age of 20 years (juvenile onset HD) occurs in approximately 5% of all HD cases.[3,4] The length of the trinucleotide repeat in HD is inversely correlated with the age of onset of the disorder.[5]
- Median survival is 24 years from diagnosis and 35 years from symptom onset (based on a sample of 5,164 individuals with HD).[6] Pneumonia, particularly aspiration pneumonia, is the most frequent cause of death, followed by other infections and suicide.[6,7]
- Motor, cognitive and psychiatric symptoms occur in HD. Chorea and dystonia are the most common movement disorders in HD. Cognitive deficits in attention, verbal fluency, psychomotor speed, executive functioning, memory and visuospatial functioning can occur in HD, even before the onset of motor symptoms.[8] Neuropsychiatric symptoms include dysphoria, agitation, irritability, apathy and anxiety.[9]

DOI: 10.4324/9781003153559-4

Background

Mary (not her real name) is 57;8 years of age. She was diagnosed with HD in 1994 when she was 34 years old. Mary has two daughters and two grandchildren, a boy and a girl. Her eldest daughter lives in Australia (she returned to live at home in September 2019). Her youngest daughter lives locally. Mary's father and two sisters died of HD. Her brother has tested positive for the HD gene **mutation**. A third sister has chosen not to be tested. Mary's eldest daughter and several of her nieces and nephews are also carriers of the HD gene.

Mary is a former deputy editor of a local newspaper. She had to stop working when she started to develop problems related to her HD. She reported that when she was "let go" from her work, she had difficulty paying her mortgage and had to rely on her daughters for financial assistance. When her youngest daughter also moved to Australia, Mary had to move out of the house she was living in and return to live in her home town. Mary currently lives on her own in a ground-floor apartment. Her youngest daughter is her official carer and she also receives substantial support from her sister. Mary sees her neurologist every six months. She does not have speech and language therapy or occupational therapy. In the past, she has had physiotherapy but found it very tiring and did not believe she received any benefit from it.

Clinical Symptoms

Mary's movements are severely affected by her HD. Her sister reports that she has involuntary "muscle spasms" (choreic movements) in her limbs, hands, feet, neck, head and body. These affect her posture, balance and **coordination**, and her ability to relax when she is sitting down. Mary is unable to stay still when she is standing. When she is walking, she finds it very difficult to keep her body upright and walk in a straight line. Because of the movements in her hands and fingers, she tends to drop things a lot.

Mary's ability to feed and swallow have also been affected by her HD. She is very nervous about choking. She used to eat liquidised food. However, she was losing weight and had to consume Fortisip (a nutritional supplement drink) and Forticreme (a semi-solid, nutritionally complete oral supplement). She then resumed normal meals and eats high-calorie foods like salmon, custard, gravy and sauces. Mary needs to concentrate when she is eating. A carer sits with her quietly during lunch and dinner. Mary feeds herself Weetabix for breakfast and takes tablets on her own at night. Mary's ability to sleep and rest are affected by her HD. Her sister describes her sleeping and rest periods as "very chaotic". Mary also has some cognitive difficulties including poor **memory** and visual-perceptual problems.

Daily Activities

All of Mary's daily activities are affected by HD. She had a car accident and is now unable to drive. She must rely on family members and friends if she wants to go out. Mary is unable to prepare meals for herself. She needs help with showering and getting dressed and undressed. She also needs help keeping up with medical appointments as she has become very forgetful. Mary used to be an avid reader. However, she does not read anymore as she finds it difficult to follow the story and remember what she has read. She likes to listen to country music and can attend concerts. She attended a concert by the American singer-songwriter Kris Kristofferson with one of her daughters. Mary enjoys watching detective programmes like *Crime Scene Investigation* and soap operas, particularly *Coronation Street* and *EastEnders*. She has made four trips to Australia to visit her eldest daughter who lived first in Brisbane and then in Melbourne. Mary has also visited Portugal. She likes to sit in the sun and get a sun tan.

Medication

Mary has been prescribed olanzapine (10 mg in the morning and evening), clonazepam (5 mg in the evening) and Circadin (2 × 2 mg). Olanzapine is used to treat psychiatric and motor symptoms in HD. Clonazepam is a benzodiazepine that is used to reduce the severity of choreic movements in HD. Circadin is used to treat insomnia.

Communication

Mary has considerable communication difficulties related to HD. Her speech has deteriorated significantly, and she now has moderately severe **dysarthria**. According to her sister, Mary's words are becoming more slurred and she often needs to repeat herself a few times to make herself understood. Mary is also struggling to use language to express herself during conversation. Her difficulties with the use of language suggest that cognitive deficits such as slowed processing and impaired **planning** may play a role in her problems. Her sister reports that Mary is finding it increasingly difficult to hold a conversation as she appears to need more time to process her thoughts and work out what she wants to say.

The author visited Mary at her home on the morning of 27 July 2018. Mary's sister was in attendance throughout the session which was conducted in the dining area of her apartment. Mary was responsive and cooperative throughout the session. Despite her significant communication difficulties, Mary was keen to communicate with the author and to undertake all tasks to the best of her ability. Her choreic movements affected her speech production and use of **gesture**. Movements of her upper body and arms made it difficult for her to attend to pictures on the table in front of her and to turn the pages in the Cinderella picture book. She wore glasses during the session and paused only to take a drink of water. She displayed no evident signs of fatigue during the session and was keen to talk further after the audio-recording was terminated. Mary showed me family photographs on her living room walls as we walked to the front door together.

Mary spoke with a creaky **voice quality**. Her **intonation** pattern and stress placement were generally good, although her speech was sometimes monotone.

There was no opportunity during the interview to assess Mary's comprehension of affective and propositional prosody, both of which are known to be impaired in HD.[10] Mary had acceptable volume and her speech was audible for the most part. Her speech rate was reduced.[11] **Fluency** was impaired on account of frequent word and phrase repetitions:[12]

> ten years of it still grand, grand and then I used to do wedding, wedding features
> she, she moved, she moved, moved to Melbourne

Mary's **articulation** of speech sounds was impaired as was her control of airflow. There was also some **hypernasality**. Problems with articulation, **respiration** and **resonance** resulted in reduced speech **intelligibility**, although there were also stretches of intelligible speech production. An unfamiliar listener assessed Mary to be 50–60% intelligible based on an audio-recording of her speech. Mary's **phonology** appeared to be reasonably intact, although a contribution from phonology to her unintelligibility cannot be excluded. Occasional errors like [stɒpwʌn] for *stopwatch* suggested she may have some phonological difficulties as well as articulatory impairments (Mary was able to produce /tʃ/ word initially, medially, and finally in *charity, Portugal* and *lunch*, respectively).

Mary displayed poor performance on the phonemic (letter) fluency task. She was only able to produce four words (*farm, fig, fir* and *fox*) beginning with the letter 'F' in 60 seconds. Moreover, she repeated the words *farm* and *fox*. Mary's **phonemic fluency** score was lower than scores obtained by both healthy individuals and by asymptomatic HD gene carriers. In one investigation, 29 people who were carriers of the HD gene obtained an average **letter fluency** score of 13.03 words. Thirty people in the same study who were not carriers of the HD gene obtained an average score of 16.32 words.[13] Mary's score was also low relative to other individuals with clinical HD.[14] In a study of phonemic fluency in 43 patients with early HD, a median of seven words beginning with the letter 'F' in 60 seconds was obtained, with a range of 0–19 words.[15]

Mary's superior semantic (category) fluency score suggests that **executive function** deficits rather than lexical access and retrieval difficulties were responsible for her poor phonemic fluency performance. That said, Mary's score of just eight animal names in 60 seconds placed her **semantic fluency** performance well below that of healthy individuals, asymptomatic HD gene carriers and individuals with clinical HD.[14] (One of her animal names, *fox*, was a possible **perseveration** from the earlier letter fluency task.) By way of comparison, asymptomatic HD gene carriers in one study produced an average of 18.12 words on the animal **category fluency** task, while people who are non-carriers obtained an average of 19.87 words.[13] In another study, the number of animal names produced by individuals with mild symptoms of HD ranged from 8 to 19 while in individuals who carried the genetic mutation but did not meet criteria for a clinical diagnosis of HD the range was 13–39.[16] Performance on category fluency tasks suggests that HD slows the retrieval of semantic memories, while **Alzheimer's disease** disrupts their storage.[17]

Deficits in **morphology** and **syntax** are reported in HD.[18,19,20] There is evidence from several languages of over-active rule processing affecting noun and verb inflections (e.g. over-suffixation as in *walkeded*).[21] Deficits in rule application are related to damage of the striatum, the key site of neurodegeneration in HD.[22,23] During picture description tasks and conversation, participants with HD produce shorter utterances, a smaller proportion of grammatical utterances, a larger proportion of simple sentences and fewer embeddings per utterance.[24,25,26]

Mary's expressive language was well-formed for the most part. She used a range of morphemes including the following inflectional and **derivational suffixes**:

the child's hair (-'*s* genitive inflectional suffix)

I stopp<u>ed</u> that (-*ed* past tense inflectional suffix)

and then obvious<u>ly</u> (-*ly* adverb derivational suffix)

detect<u>ive</u> stories (-*ive* derivational suffix)

I was a report<u>er</u> (-*er* derivational suffix)

print<u>ing</u> department (-*ing* derivational suffix)

Mary also used a range of grammatical structures, including relative and **infinitive clauses, passive voice** constructions and negation:

ugly sisters <u>who were cruel to her</u>

(relative clause)

we were going <u>to go last November</u>

(infinitive clause)

I <u>was let go</u>

(passive voice)

I could<u>n't</u> pay the mortgage

(negation)

The comprehension of logico-grammatically complex sentences, including passive voice sentences, is reported to be impaired in people with HD.[25]

During conversation about her previous employment, Mary used a syntactic construction called **topicalisation**. In the second utterance below, the **noun phrase** *Jan Fleming* (not her real name) is a **subject complement**. It is fronted in this sentence to allow Mary to place emphasis on the identity of the editor:

> This new managing editor come into the building. Jan Fleming her name was

However, Mary also abandoned many utterances at midpoint, leaving sentences with incomplete structure. For example, she abandoned the following utterance before she completed the **subordinate clause**:

> nobody realised that I had a, you know only when I talked to family

Phrases were also abandoned such as the incomplete **verb phrases** in the following utterances:

> rarely buying them cause I couldn't, I couldn't, I was eating breakfast Weetabix
> she's not allowing, but then her godmother come

During these abandoned utterances, Mary appeared to lose the thread of what she wanted to say. This suggests a problem with **planning** her utterances and is consistent with the observation of Mary's sister that Mary needed more time to process her thoughts and work out what she wanted to say.

Mary had considerable lexical-semantic impairments. During **confrontation naming**, she named only 6 of 18 pictures correctly, a finding that replicates earlier reports of poor performance on visual confrontation naming.[27-29] The remaining 12 pictures were named following the use of cues. The cues used to elicit target words were semantic, phonemic and gestural in nature. For example, Mary successfully named 'nose' when she was given the **semantic cue** *it's part of your face*. Occasionally, a cue was misunderstood and led to incorrect naming of a picture. This occurred when the author mimed playing an accordion only for Mary to produce the word *trombone*. Also, the semantic cue for 'seahorse' triggered the related word *dolphin*. Visual-perceptual errors are commonly reported in HD.[27,30] They tended to dominate during Mary's naming, as the following examples illustrate:

'crown' → container of broccoli
'ostrich' → giraffe
'pumpkin' → onion/tomato
'thimble' → it's like a vase
'lobster' → something with ears ('ears' used to describe pincers)

Even as Mary excluded certain answers during her naming, it was clear that visual-perceptual difficulties were again evident. For example, for 'whistle' Mary responded *it's not a mobile phone*, and for 'accordion' she said *it's not a suitcase*.

Other errors appeared to be semantic in nature:

'duck' → *stork*

'train' → *bus wagon*

'spanner' → *screwdriver*

Lexical-semantic errors were occasionally evident during spontaneous conversation and other types of **discourse** production. Mary produced words that were semantically related to their targets, such as the use of *rent* for 'mortgage' during conversation:

> to help me with the rent, the rent and I couldn't pay the mortgage

There was little evidence of word-finding difficulties in Mary's conversation. What is clear, however, is that visual-perceptual deficits played a significant role in Mary's lexical choices during discourse production and resulted in misrepresentations of people and actions in pictures. In the Cookie Theft picture, for example, the mother was drying dishes and not doing the child's hair:

> her mother is doing the child hair, hair

Visual-perceptual deficits were also responsible for some of Mary's lexical errors during the Flowerpot Incident. In the first picture in the sequence, Mary erroneously described the balcony as a wardrobe and the falling flowerpot as a light. The man who is crouching in pain after being struck by the flowerpot was described as a child sitting down:

> it seems to be a wardrobe, and em, it's sitting, sitting down, child is sitting down, nearer the wardrobe and there's a light above them

Another lexical error during the Flowerpot Incident was the use of the word *bureau*. This was a **perseveration** from the previous task where Mary was asked to generate a sentence that contained the words *bureau, open* and *drawer*.

Both the Cookie Theft picture and the Flowerpot Incident narrative involve considerable action verb language such as the boy is *falling* off the stool, the man is *banging* the door of the apartment, and the man is *walking* along the street with his dog. None of this language is used by Mary. People with HD have been found to produce fewer action information units than healthy individuals during picture description.[31] They are also reported to have a deficit in verb production, the latter related to a disorder of the motor loop in HD speakers with **dementia**.[28]

Mary displayed an understanding of lexical relations between words. During confrontation naming, she was struggling to name a picture of a *nose*. The author provided two semantic cues. The first cue took the form of a question 'Do you think it might be something *on your face*?' Mary responded with *glasses* in response to this cue. A follow-up cue from the author was more specific about the relationship of the target word to a face at which point Mary responded with *nose*. This revealed that Mary had an appreciation of the part–whole relation of meronymy between the words *nose* (part) and *face* (whole):

INV: here's a clue, do you think it might be something on your face? Does it remind you of something on your face?
MAR: um aye gla, not glasses
INV: part of your face
MAR: oh, your nose

Mary displayed good understanding of sentence meaning and was able to construct meaningful utterances for the most part. During sentence generation, she constructed not only well-formed sentences but also sentences that were meaningful. The utterance she produced for the word *tree* displayed an appropriate use of the conditional meaning of the **subordinating conjunction** *if*:

the tree can be green or brown if it's autumn

For the words *chair*, *doctor* and *sit*, there was some inconsistency in Mary's use of locative **prepositions** to represent spatial relations. While in terms of their **semantics** either *in* or *on* is acceptable in front of *chair*, only *in* can be used before *doctor's*:

we sit in, on the chair up on the doctor's

Mary displayed intact use and understanding of several pragmatic features of language. The comprehension of **figurative language** has been found to be impaired in HD.[32],[33] Mary was able to understand one form of figurative language – idiomatic language – when it was used by the author:

INV: so, a future trip to Australia is *on the cards*

Mary also made context-appropriate use of idiomatic language:

MAR: the family *hadn't the heart to* tell me

Deictic expressions were used extensively by Mary. In this example of **discourse deixis**, the **demonstrative pronoun** *that* referred to Mary's earlier account of attending the Kris Kristofferson concert with her daughter Megan:

I was at Kris Kristofferson wasn't I in Belfast, in Belfast me and me daughter went Megan so <u>that</u> was brilliant

Mary used spatial deixis in the form of the **adverb** *here* to explain the problems she experienced with feeding and swallowing when she first moved into her apartment:

> I was, I was on liquidised food for a while when I come <u>here</u> first

There was evidence that Mary was able to undertake **conversational repair** of her utterances. She used self-initiated self-repair in several **discourse** contexts:

> butter the bread and then put butter, put mayonnaise on
>
> *(procedural discourse)*

> then the editor would write, read them back
>
> *(conversation)*

Mary also appreciated **humour** in conversation and made context-appropriate use of laughter, as illustrated by the following exchange:

INV: I now need to get my stopwatch in to (.) so (.) this is a museum piece *(laughter)* have you ever seen an older mobile phone?
MAR: *(laughter)*

Mary used some forms of **cohesion** to good effect. This included grammatical **ellipsis:** as in the following exchange:

MAR: she's still trying to get another baby
INV: right, okay, well I'm sure that'll work out for her
MAR: it will, it will

In the exchange below, Mary uses the **pronoun** *it* to refer to her decision to resume eating ordinary meals:

> I stopped that I put on ordinary <u>taking ordinary meal</u> but ah still I don't I still don't do <u>it</u> on my own, if you know what I mean

Alongside these strengths in **pragmatics** and **discourse** were some areas of weakness. Mary was often repetitive in her use of language. During the Flowerpot Incident, she states twice that the man is taking the dog for a walk:

> there's umbrella the girl or the man um somebody with a hat is with umbrella aye at the wardrobe aye and taking the dog possibly for a walk (.) puppy and then the child the person aye again the dog, um the dog erm her again the woman and man (.) are at the door (.) and again must be taking the dog possibly for a walk

Mary was also repetitive on occasions in conversation. In the following exchange, she repeats the fact that her daughter moved to Melbourne. Additionally, she appears to convey contradictory information, first by saying that her grandson was born *before* her daughter moved to Melbourne and then stating that he was born *after* she moved to Melbourne:

> when she had a wee child XXX [*grandson's name*] she moved to Melbourne em due to, to be with my family me niece and nephew aye so she, she moved, she moved, moved to Melbourne and then XXX [*grandson's name*] was born there

Mary frequently omitted information during narration and picture description. Her description of the Cookie Theft picture omits several key details: the mother is drying the dishes; the sink is overflowing with water; and the boy is about to fall off the stool. So much information was omitted from Mary's telling of the Cinderella story that it bore little resemblance to the original tale.

Other pragmatic and discourse difficulties included some insensitivity to the listener's knowledge state, as evidenced by Mary's use of the names of acquaintances who were not known to the author and had not been introduced earlier in the conversation:

> I bought the CD loved it, loved it and <u>Pat</u> paid
> <u>Mark</u> was away, he worked in the mines you see

Mary's use of proper nouns to refer to people who are not part of the wider discourse context is consistent with the finding that people with pre-symptomatic HD have problems with the referential use of language to identify characters in a story.[34]

During Cinderella narration, Mary appeared to assume that the author would be able to identify the **referent** of the **pronoun** *they* when she had not established a referent for this pronoun in the prior discourse context:

> <u>they</u> knew it was the old shoe not the em, not the beautiful shoe

Mary's insensitivity to listener knowledge raised the possibility that she had some difficulty establishing the mental states of others, that is, a problem with **theory of mind** (ToM). A possible ToM deficit was also suggested by the fact that Mary did not use mental state language to capture the cognitive and **affective mental states** of characters in stories or during picture description. For example, Mary did not mention that the mother in the Cookie Theft picture was *daydreaming* and had *forgotten* to turn off the tap, or that the man in the Flowerpot Incident was *angry* that he had been struck on the head by a falling flowerpot. The omission of these mental states is consistent with the ToM deficits that are known to occur in HD.[35,36] As well as having a specific deficit in the recognition of negative emotions such as anger, disgust and fear,[35,37] people with HD have also been found to be impaired in recognising emotional body language[38] and angry whole-body postures in particular.[39] It is noteworthy that Mary failed to attribute any significance to the angry body posture of the man in the Flowerpot Incident.

Finally, while Mary was skilled in the use of some **presuppositions**, there was evidence that presuppositions were not always used appropriately by her. She used the change-of-state verb *start* during conversation which triggers the presupposition that a certain action (in this case, interviewing) had not previously taken place. But she then immediately overrides that presupposition by stating that she used to be interviewed. Her utterance is pragmatically anomalous as a result:

> she <u>started</u> interviewing me and she used to interview me about why my stories weren't long enough

COMMUNICATION PROFILE:

Speech intelligibility:

- Mary's speech intelligibility is reduced, due to dysarthria; her voice quality is 'creaky'; articulation is compromised by impaired control of airflow. Mary is audible in a conversation conducted in a quiet setting. Her speech rate is reduced and her fluency impaired. Mary's intonation and stress are quite good although there is also some monotonous speech. Phonology may be a contributory factor to Mary's unintelligibility.

Morphology and syntax:

- Mary's use of inflectional and derivational morphemes is intact. She varies her syntactic structures to include relative and infinitive clauses, passive voice constructions, negation and topicalisation. Syntax may be incomplete due to abandonment of utterances; Mary shows good comprehension of grammar in conversation

Vocabulary and semantics:

- Mary exhibits visual-perceptual and semantic deficits during confrontation naming; visual-perceptual errors in lexical use in discourse; poor semantic fluency; no evident word-finding difficulty in conversation although occasional semantic errors and lexical perseveration did occur; good understanding of lexical relations; subordinating conjunctions are used meaningfully in sentences but there is some inconsistency in use of locative prepositions.

Pragmatics:

-   Mary uses and understands idiomatic language; has good use of deixis; can participate in conversational repair; appreciates humour and makes context-appropriate use of laughter; and uses a range of presuppositions with occasional errors.

Discourse:

-   Mary uses ellipsis and pronominal reference effectively as cohesive devices. She repeats, omits and conveys contradictory information in discourse and is insensitive to listener knowledge when she uses proper names and pronouns without referents. Mary does not use mental state language of protagonists in stories and pictures.

Cognition:

-   Mary's significant executive function deficits are suggested by her poor phonemic fluency, and reports of slowed information processing and poor planning in conversation. ToM deficits are suggested by a lack of mental state language and difficulty establishing listener knowledge.

Suggestions for Further Reading

(1)   Quarrell, O. (2008) *Huntington's Disease,* Second Edition. Oxford: Oxford University Press.

This volume contains 12 chapters on all aspects of HD, including basic facts and figures about the disorder, its physical, behavioural and emotional features, genetics and neuropathology. There is also a dedicated chapter on juvenile HD. A glossary of key terms is available.

(2)   Hamilton, A., Ferm, U., Heemskerk, A.-W., Twiston-Davies, R., Matheson, K.Y., Simpson, S.A., Rae, D. and On behalf of the contributing members of the European Huntington's Disease Networks Standards of Care Speech and Language Therapist Group. (2012) 'Management of speech, language and communication difficulties in Huntington's disease', *Neurodegenerative Disease Management,* 2 (1): 67–77.

This article comprehensively examines the management of communication problems in individuals with HD. It is written by expert speech and language therapists from across Europe who were tasked with producing guidelines for the management of communication disorders in HD by the European Huntington's Disease Network Standards of Care Speech and Language Therapy Working Group.

(3) Bayles, K. and Tomoeda, C.K. (2013) *Cognitive-Communication Disorders of Dementia: Definition, Diagnosis, and Treatment,* Second Edition. San Diego, CA: Plural Publishing.

Chapter 9 in this book examines the genetics, neuropathology and symptomatology of HD. The latter includes affect and motor symptoms, and the effects of HD on speech, language, communication and cognition. The chapter is a comprehensive treatment of the effect of HD on all aspects of communication.

Questions

(1) Mary displayed several pragmatic language skills during conversation and other forms of discourse. She was able to understand indirect speech acts when these were used by the author. For the most part, she used presuppositions appropriately. She was able to undertake self-initiated self-repair in conversation. Mary also made effective use of ellipsis to achieve cohesion in discourse and used several forms of deixis. Five of Mary's utterances are shown below. Identify the pragmatic language skill exemplified by each of these utterances:

(a) "I used to drive but I stopped driving"
(b) "I would have gone to the court, council meetings in the evening"
(c) INV: Can you tell me about your previous employment? MAR: I was a reporter
(d) "we were going to go last November but then she lost the baby"
(e) INV: So, you were reporting on court cases? MAR: I was indeed, I was indeed

(2) Mary was asked by the author to describe how she would make a ham and cheese sandwich. Examine the steps she outlined, and then answer the questions below:

MAR: well in I don't like toast, so I'd be making bread
INV: okay
MAR: bre, bread butter, butter the bread and then put butter, put mayonnaise on
INV: okay
MAR: so something time, and ham did you say?
INV: yes, ham and cheese
MAR: aye ham so you'd be ah taking out the slice of ham from, from cupboard and then cheese also you'd slice and then um erm you'd get then in you'd put it in again cut it cut them into [pɔrk peɪs pleɪsɪz] cut pieces

(a) This extract contains the only question that Mary posed during the entire session with the author. What purpose does this question serve?

(b) Does Mary make any lexical-semantic errors during her account of sandwich making?

(c) Does Mary use canonical (S-V-O) word order?

(d) Does Mary construct the discourse context in a way that allows the listener to establish the referents of the pronouns she uses?

(e) Towards the end of her account, Mary says "put it in *again*". What presupposition is triggered by *again*?

(3) Some of Mary's utterances contained missing, contradictory or erroneous information and were difficult for the hearer to follow. Five examples of this type of utterance are shown below. Identify the problem source in each utterance:

[*Note*: 'be's on' in (b) and 'me own', 'me tablets' and 'me custard' in (e) are grammatical features of Mary's dialect of English.]

(a) "I bought the CD loved it, loved it and Pat paid"

(b) "there's a wee programme 5USA that be's on erm not too sure what station anyway it be's on the NCIS"

(c) "when I come here first and bought, bought no I think rarely buying them cause I couldn't, I couldn't, I was eating breakfast Weetabix"

(d) In response to a question about which TV programmes she likes, Mary proceeds to say she likes any of the soaps: "I know ah sure any of them, em the wee soaps *EastEnders* you know any of them *EastEnders*, I don't really like *Emmerdale*"

(e) "I will never eat on me own. I have ah breakfast Weetabix in the morning here try, try to eat and even take, take me tablets at night I take me custard have so that on me own"

(4) During confrontation naming, cues were not always effective in prompting Mary to produce the target word. Examine the following naming responses and describe the type of cues that elicited or failed to elicit the target word in each case:

(a) Target 'ostrich': initial response *giraffe*, followed by cue: 'do you think it might be any type of bird?' Second response *turkey*. Additional cue: 'this bird runs quite fast and we can also eat it, not commonly, but we do sometimes eat the meat of this bird'. Third response *reindeer*.

(b) Target 'whistle': initial response *not a mobile phone*, followed by cue: 'I might use this if I was out on the playing field, with refereeing a hockey match or football match or something like that'. Second response *stopwatch*. Additional cue: 'I might blow into it, it's a wh..'. Third response *whistle*.

(c) Target 'accordion': initial response *not a suitcase*, followed by cue: 'it's a type of musical instrument and you see people playing it by pushing and pulling it in and out like this [*mimes playing accordion*]'. Second response *trombone*. Third response *piano*. Additional cue: 'it's ack ... if you were playing it you would move it in and out like this'. Fourth response *accordion*.

(d) Target 'thimble': initial response *it's like a vase*, followed by cue: 'do you do needle work? You might use this on your fingers and thumbs. It begins with th ...'. Second response *thumb*. Third response *thimble*.

Answers

(1) (a) presupposition (*stopped* is a change–of–state verb that triggers the pre-supposition that Mary used to drive)
   (b) self-initiated, self-repair
   (c) indirect speech act (a request)
   (d) temporal deixis (*last* November)
   (e) ellipsis (I was indeed [*reporting on court cases*])
(2) (a) When Mary asks "ham, did you say?", she is checking the accuracy of her recall of the task instruction.
   (b) Mary uses *cupboard* when the word 'fridge' is more appropriate for the storage of ham.
   (c) Mary does not use canonical word order when she says, "cheese also you'd slice". This is O-S-V word order.
   (d) Mary does not construct a discourse context that would allow her lis-tener to establish the referents of the pronouns she uses. The pronoun *it* in "put it" and "cut it" could refer to cheese or the sandwich. There is no identifiable referent of *them* in "cut them".
   (e) The iterative expression *again* triggers the presupposition that 'it' had been 'put in' *before*.
(3) (a) Mary says that she bought the CD (that is, *paid* for it) only to then say that Pat paid for it. Her utterance contains contradictory information.
   (b) Mary is confusing a channel (5USA) with a programme (NCIS: Naval Criminal Investigative Service). Her utterance contains erroneous information.
   (c) Mary states that she bought 'them' (presumably, Weetabix) only to then say that she rarely bought them. She then proceeds to explain why she rarely bought Weetabix but omits the very information that would con-vey her reason. Her utterance contains contradictory information and omits information.
   (d) Mary begins by saying she likes *any* of the soaps only to then say she does *not* like *Emmerdale*. Her utterance contains contradictory information.
   (e) Mary begins by saying that she *never* eats on her own. She then goes on to say that she takes tablets and food (Weetabix and custard) on her own. Her utterance contains contradictory information.

(4) (a) Two semantic cues are ineffective in eliciting production of the target word.

     (b) Initially, a semantic cue fails to elicit production of the target word. Then, another semantic cue followed by a phonemic cue succeeds in eliciting the target word.

     (c) Initially, a semantic cue followed by a gestural cue (mime) fails to elicit production of the target word. Then, a phonemic cue followed by the same mime (gestural cue) succeeds in eliciting the target word.

     (d) A semantic cue followed by a phonemic cue fails to elicit the target word initially. However, without further cuing, Mary then succeeds in producing the target word.

References

[1] McColgan, P. and Tabrizi, S.J. (2018) 'Huntington's disease: A clinical review', *European Journal of Neurology*, 25 (1): 24–34.

[2] Pringsheim, T., Wiltshire, K., Day, L., Dykeman, J., Steeves, T. and Jette, N. (2012) 'The incidence and prevalence of Huntington's disease: A systematic review and meta-analysis', *Movement Disorders*, 27 (9): 1083–1091.

[3] Bhidayasiri, R. and Tarsy, D. (2012) *Movement Disorders: A Video Atlas. Current Clinical Neurology.* Totowa, NJ: Humana Press.

[4] Quarrell, O., O'Donovan, K.L., Bandmann, O. and Strong, M. (2012) 'The prevalence of juvenile Huntington's disease: A review of the literature and meta-analysis', *PLoS Currents*, 4: e4f8606b742ef3.

[5] Duyao, M., Ambrose, C., Myers, R., Novelletto, A., Persichetti, F., Frontali, M., Folstein, S., Ross, C., Franz, M., Abbott, M., et al. (1993) 'Trinucleotide repeat length instability and age of onset in Huntington's disease', *Nature Genetics*, 4 (4): 387–392.

[6] Rodrigues, F.B., Abreu, D., Damásio, J., Gonçalves, N., Correia-Guedes, L., Coelho, M., Ferreira, J.J. and REGISTRY Investigators of the European Huntington's Disease Network (2017) 'Survival, mortality, causes and places of death in a European Huntington's disease prospective cohort', *Movement Disorders*, 4 (5): 737–742.

[7] Heemskerk, A.-W. and Roos, R.A.C. (2012) 'Aspiration pneumonia and death in Huntington's disease', *PLoS Currents Huntington Disease*. Edition 1. doi:10.1371/currents.RRN1293.

[8] Duff, K., Paulsen, J., Mills, J., Beglinger, L.J., Moser, D.J., Smith, M.M., Langbehn, D., Stout, J., Queller, S., Harrington, D.L., and on behalf of the PREDICT-HD Investigators and Coordinators of the Huntington Study Group (2010) 'Mild cognitive impairment in prediagnosed Huntington disease', *Neurology*, 75 (6): 500–507.

[9] Paulsen, J., Ready, R., Hamilton, J., Mega, M. and Cummings, J. (2001) 'Neuropsychiatric aspects of Huntington's disease', *Journal of Neurology, Neurosurgery & Psychiatry*, 71 (3): 310–314.

[10] Speedie, L.J., Brake, N., Folstein, S.E., Bowers, D. and Heilman, K.M. (1990) 'Comprehension of prosody in Huntington's disease', *Journal of Neurology, Neurosurgery, and Psychiatry*, 53 (7): 607–610.

[11] Skodda, S., Schlegel, U., Hoffmann, R. and Saft, C. (2014) 'Impaired motor speech performance in Huntington's disease', *Journal of Neural Transmission*, 121 (4): 399–407.

[12] Tovar, A., Soler, A.G., Ruiz-Idiago, J., Viladrich, C.M., Pomarol-Clotet, E., Roselló, J. and Hinzen, W. (2020) 'Language disintegration in spontaneous speech in Huntington's disease: A more fine-grained analysis', *Journal of Communication Disorders*, 83: 105970.

[13] Larsson, M.U., Almkvist, O., Luszcz, M.A. and Wahlin, T.B. (2008) 'Phonemic fluency deficits in asymptomatic gene carriers for Huntington's disease', *Neuropsychology*, 22 (5): 596–605.

[14] Rosser, A. and Hodges, J.R. (1994) 'Initial letter and semantic category fluency in Alzheimer's disease, Huntington's disease, and progressive supranuclear palsy', *Journal of Neurology, Neurosurgery & Psychiatry*, 57 (11): 1389–1394.

[15] Snowden, J.S., Craufurd, D., Thompson, J. and Neary, D. (2002) 'Psychomotor, executive, and memory function in preclinical Huntington's disease', *Journal of Clinical and Experimental Neuropsychology*, 24 (2): 133–145.

[16] Júlio, F., Ribeiro, M.J., Patrício, M., Malhão, A., Pedrosa, F., Gonçalves, H., Simões, M., van Asselen, M., Simões, M.R., Castelo-Branco, M. and Januário, C. (2019) 'A novel ecological approach reveals early executive function impairments in Huntington's disease', *Frontiers in Psychology*, 10: 585. doi: 10.3389/fpsyg.2019.00585.

[17] Rohrer, D., Salmon, D.P., Wixted, J.T. and Paulsen, J.S. (1999) 'The disparate effects of Alzheimer's disease and Huntington's disease on semantic memory', *Neuropsychology*, 13 (3): 381–388.

[18] Gagnon, M., Barrette, J. and Macoir, J. (2018) 'Language disorders in Huntington disease: A systematic literature review', *Cognitive and Behavioral Neurology*, 31 (4): 179–192.

[19] Illes, J. (1989) 'Neurolinguistic features of spontaneous language production dissociate three forms of neurodegenerative disease: Alzheimer's, Huntington's, and Parkinson's', *Brain and Language*, 37 (4): 628–642.

[20] García, A.M., Bocanegra, Y., Herrera, E., Pino, M., Muñoz, E., Sedeño, L. and Ibáñez, A. (2018) 'Action-semantic and syntactic deficits in subjects at risk for Huntington's disease', *Journal of Neuropsychology*, 12 (3): 389–408.

[21] Nemeth, D. Dye, C.D., Sefcsik, T., Janacsek, K., Turi, Z., Londe, Z., Klivenyi, P., Kincses, Z.T., Szabó, N., Vecsei, L. and Ullman, M.T. (2012) 'Language deficits in presymptomatic Huntington's disease: Evidence from Hungarian', *Brain and Language*, 121 (3): 248–253.

[22] Teichmann, M., Gaura, V., Démonet, J.-F., Supiot, F., Delliaux, M., Verny, C., Renou, P., Remy, P. and Bachoud-Lévi, A.-C. (2008) 'Language processing within the striatum: Evidence from a PET correlation study in Huntington's disease', *Brain*, 131 (4): 1046–1056.

[23] Teichmann, M., Dupoux, E., Kouider, S. and Bachoud-Lévi, A.-C. (2006) 'The role of the striatum in processing language rules: Evidence from word perception in Huntington's disease', *Journal of Cognitive Neuroscience*, 18 (9): 1555–1569.

[24] Murray, L.L. (2000) 'Spoken language production in Huntington's and Parkinson's diseases', *Journal of Speech, Language, and Hearing Research*, 43 (6): 1350–1366.

[25] Gordon, W.P. and Illes, J. (1987) 'Neurolinguistic characteristics of language production in Huntington's disease: A preliminary report', *Brain and Language*, 31 (1): 1–10.

[26] Murray, L.L. and Lenz, L.P. (2001) 'Productive syntax abilities in Huntington's and Parkinson's diseases', *Brain and Cognition*, 46 (1–2): 213–219.

[27] Podoll, K., Caspary, P., Lange, H.W. and Noth, J. (1988) 'Language functions in Huntington's disease', *Brain*, 111 (6): 1475–1503.

[28] Péran, P., Démonet, J.-F., Pernet, C. and Cardebat, D. (2004) 'Verb and noun generation tasks in Huntington's disease', *Movement Disorders*, 19 (5): 565–571.

[29] Wallesch, C.W. and Fehrenbach, R.A. (1988) 'On the neurolinguistic nature of language abnormalities in Huntington's disease', *Journal of Neurology, Neurosurgery, and Psychiatry*, 51 (3): 367–373.

[30] Hodges, J.R., Salmon, D.P. and Butlers, N. (1991) 'The nature of the naming deficit in Alzheimer's and Huntington's disease', *Brain*, 114 (4): 1547–1558.

[31] Jensen, A.M., Chenery, H.J. and Copland, D.A. (2006) 'A comparison of picture description abilities in individuals with vascular subcortical lesions and Huntington's disease', *Journal of Communication Disorders*, 39 (1): 62–77.

[32] Saldert, C., Fors, A., Ströberg, S. and Hartelius, L. (2010) 'Comprehension of complex discourse in different stages of Huntington's disease', *International Journal of Language & Communication Disorders*, 45 (6): 656–669.

[33] Chenery, H.J., Copland, D.A. and Murdoch, B.E. (2002) 'Complex language functions and subcortical mechanisms: Evidence from Huntington's disease and patients with non-thalamic subcortical lesions', *International Journal of Language and Communication Disorders*, 37 (4): 459–474.

[34] Hinzen, W., Rosselló, J., Morey, C., Camara, E., Garcia-Gorro, C., Salvador, R. and de Diego-Balaguer, R. (2018) 'A systematic linguistic profile of spontaneous narrative speech in pre-symptomatic and early stage Huntington's disease', *Cortex*, 100: 71–83.

[35] Bora, E., Velakoulis, D. and Walterfang, M. (2016) 'Social cognition in Huntington's disease: A meta-analysis', *Behavioural Brain Research*, 297: 131–140.

[36] Larsen, I.U., Vinther-Jensen, T., Gade, A., Nielsen, J.E. and Vogel, A. (2016) 'Do I misconstrue? Sarcasm detection, emotion recognition, and theory of mind in Huntington disease', *Neuropsychology*, 30 (2): 181–189.

[37] Hayes, C.J., Stevenson, R.J. and Coltheart, M. (2007) 'Disgust and Huntington's disease', *Neuropsychologia*, 45 (6): 1135–1151.

[38] Zarotti, N., Fletcher, I. and Simpson, J. (2019) 'New perspectives on emotional processing in people with symptomatic Huntington's disease: Impaired emotion regulation and recognition of emotional body language', *Archives of Clinical Neuropsychology*, 34 (5): 610–624.

[39] De Gelder, B., Van den Stock, J., de Diego-Balaguer, R. and Bachoud-Lévi, A.-C. (2008) 'Huntington's disease impairs recognition of angry and instrumental body language', *Neuropsychologia*, 46 (1): 369–373.

CASE STUDY 4

Lewy Body Disease

KEY FACTS AND FIGURES:

- Lewy body disease (LBD) is a progressive degenerative brain disorder in which clusters of alpha-synuclein protein called 'Lewy bodies' accumulate inside and outside neurons. Neurons that produce the neurotransmitter dopamine are particularly vulnerable to the accumulation of Lewy bodies.
- The prevalence of LBD varies significantly across studies. LBD prevalence ranged from 2.4% to 5.9% in nine secondary care services in two English regions.[1] A systematic review of prevalence studies reported that prevalence estimates ranged from 0% to 5% of the general population, and from 0% to 30.5% of all dementia cases.[2] The incidence rate varies with country of study: 3.5 per 100,000 person-years in the USA and 7.10 per 100,000 person-years in Taiwan.[3,4] Women and men develop LBD in roughly equal numbers (the female: male sex ratio in one French sample of 10,309 individuals was 1.21: 1).[5] Prevalence and incidence figures should be interpreted against a backdrop of considerable under-diagnosis of LBD.
- Risk factors for LBD include advanced age, male sex, a family history of dementia, depression and low caffeine intake.[6]
- Core clinical features include recurrent visual hallucinations,[7,8,9] cognitive fluctuations, REM sleep behaviour disorder,[10] and one or more cardinal features of Parkinsonism (bradykinesia, rest tremor or rigidity). Other symptoms include delusions (e.g. of other people stealing),[11] olfactory dysfunction,[12] seizures and myoclonus.[13]

DOI: 10.4324/9781003153559-5

- Age of onset is typically between 50 and 85 years of age. The average survival time from diagnosis in a pooled sample of 2,029 patients with dementia with Lewy bodies was 4.11 years.[14] Median survival time is approximately 4.0 years.[15,16] In a survey of 658 carers and family members of individuals with LBD, causes of death were reported to be failure to thrive (65%), followed by pneumonia and swallowing difficulties (23%), other medical conditions (19%) and complications from falling (10%).[17]

Background

Thomas (not his real name) is 56;6 years old. He is married with three children (two sons and a daughter) from his first marriage and three stepchildren (two stepsons and a stepdaughter) from his second marriage. Thomas, his wife and all six of their children left their home country over a period of several years and moved to Australia. Thomas and his wife have since returned home after spending five years in Australia. On 11 September 2017, Thomas' neurologist informed him that he had LBD. He was 54 years old at the time. This superseded an earlier diagnosis of **Parkinson's disease**. Thomas no longer works. When he was employed, he worked in construction and sales. He owned his own building company and a fitted furniture company. He has worked as a site manager of an apartment block and has designed and sold kitchens, bedroom units, wardrobes and shower screens. Thomas has enjoyed all the jobs he has had over the years although he found self-employment very stressful. He has a university diploma in psychology. Thomas' maternal uncle was diagnosed with Lewy body dementia and may have had previous Parkinsonism. His paternal uncle was diagnosed with Alzheimer's dementia.

Thomas has had many hospitalisations and episodes of ill health as an adult. In the early 1980s, he had knee surgery for a sports injury that resulted in damaged cartilage. He was in a full cast from his groin to his ankle for six weeks. In 1995, during a visit to Jersey to see his brother, Thomas took a boat and bus trip to a little market in the north of France. During this trip, he experienced a "weird reverberation" inside his brain. Suddenly, he was unable to see or walk properly, or communicate with anyone. He did not mention this episode to his brother and did not seek medical assistance. His second hospitalisation occurred in 1999 when he had an operation for a prolapsed disc. Although his keyhole surgery was successful, he did not follow medical advice on his recovery time and ended up back in hospital twice within a couple of months having two separate epidurals in his back to relieve severe pain.

Thomas was diagnosed with high blood pressure in 2002 and has had several episodes of chest pain and breathing difficulties. In July 2013, he developed

Coxsackie virus, an infection he contracted from babysitting his grandson who had hand, foot and mouth disease. In October 2014, Thomas was hospitalised when he developed viral **meningitis**. While he was recovering in hospital, medical staff became aware that he had pain when trying to get out of bed. A nuclear bone scan was performed, and Thomas was diagnosed with Paget's disease of the bone. In January 2015, Thomas was hospitalised for one week when he contracted the H1N1 virus. In 2016, he was diagnosed with diverticulitis and asthma. Thomas was diagnosed with cervical **spinal stenosis** in August 2019. He also has obstructive **sleep apnoea** and uses a continuous positive airway pressure (CPAP) machine at night to alleviate his breathing difficulties. Although he does not smoke now, Thomas smoked around 20 cigarettes a day for approximately 20 years. He stopped drinking alcohol in 1990 and was teetotal for 11 years.

Thomas has had a long and arduous road to diagnosis of LBD. On 6 October 2015, he had a neurological examination. His consultant neurologist reported that **cranial nerves** II to XII were intact. His peripheral nerve exam showed no abnormalities and his gait was normal. His **Romberg test** was negative. Thomas displayed mild **ataxia** while sitting with his eyes closed. No **cerebellar signs** were present. The neurologist performed a **lumbar puncture** on 13 November 2015. The **cerebrospinal fluid** (CSF) was negative for pathological Tau protein. Serum protein electrophoresis (SPEP) was negative for **oligoclonal bands** in the serum and CSF.

A further neurological examination was conducted on 8 March 2016. Again, cranial nerves II to XII were intact with no sensory or motor deficit. Thomas had truncal ataxia and difficulty with **tandem gait**. There was decreased swing of his right arm and resting **tremor** of his left arm with **cogwheeling** evidence bilaterally. There was no **hypomimia**. Thomas had a negative **past pointing test**. There was no intention tremor and no **rebound**. On examination of the peripheral nervous system, Thomas had brisk reflexes in both lower limbs. **Clonus** was evident in the left lower limb with 67 beats and clonus in the right lower limb was sustained. Plantars were downgoing. Thomas' STOP-Bang score was 8/8 (high risk for moderate to severe obstructive sleep apnoea) and his Epworth Sleepiness Scale score was 14/24 (moderate excessive daytime sleepiness). A week later, on 15 March 2016, a brain PET CT was conducted. The findings were normal.

Thomas was told he would have a follow-up appointment in March 2017. When this did not come about, he contacted the hospital, to be informed that it would be several months before he would receive an appointment. Thomas' doctor wrote to his neurologist in March 2017, stating that Thomas was anxious to have an appointment as early as possible.

On 1 June 2017, Thomas was again seen as an outpatient by his neurologist. At this assessment, his copying of a spiral drawing was very irregular (see Figure 4.1). He was observed to walk with a small step and a reduced left arm swing. He displayed rest tremor on the left arm when he walked. There was no freezing and no shuffling. Thomas had some difficulty in turning around. He had a negative

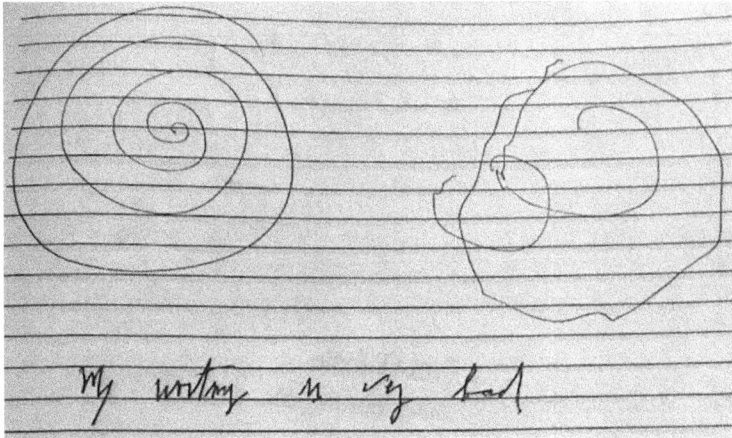

FIGURE 4.1   Sample of Thomas' writing and copying spiral drawing, 27 February 2018. It was very difficult for Thomas to write but his writing did not display micrographia.

retropulsion test. There was **bradykinesia** mainly affecting the right leg and upper limbs bilaterally. Thomas had mild **rigidity** on the left upper limb and normal tone on the right. His eye movement was normal and there were no cerebellar or **pyramidal signs**. On 16 August 2017, a nuclear medicine dopamine active transfer scan (NM DAT scan) was conducted. It was compared with the normal PET CT conducted on 15 March 2016. It revealed relatively decreased uptake in the right caudate head compared with the left, suggesting an early dopaminergic deficit. The radiologist concluded that the findings supported a diagnosis of a true Parkinsonian syndrome. Thomas' neurologist diagnosed **idiopathic Parkinson's disease** or **Parkinson's plus syndrome** such as LBD.

Clinical Symptoms

Given the protracted nature of Thomas' health problems, it is difficult to discern which of his many symptoms of illness are directly related to LBD (see Table 4.1). Approximately six months before his diagnosis of LBD, Thomas reported experiencing hip pain, blurred vision, slurred speech, poor handwriting, sudden sweating, confusion, tremors, stopping mid-sentence, reduced appetite, intolerance of loud noise, as well as other symptoms (viz., diverticulitis, asthma and fluctuating energy levels).

Thomas suffers from **REM sleep behaviour disorder**. He has vivid, terrifying nightmares that are all about murder, death and mayhem: "There are days when all that I can think about are the nightmares from the night before and I can get so caught up in them that before I know it my day has gone, and the cycle starts all over again." These nightmares have increased in frequency with

TABLE 4.1 Thomas' range of symptoms according to his wife

Physical symptoms	Psychiatric symptoms
Blood pressure	Anxiety
Chest pain	Depression
Dizziness	Delusion
Drowsiness	Delirium
Excessive daytime sleepiness	Suicidal thoughts
Insomnia	Visual hallucinations
Kidney infections	
Nausea	
Night sweats	
Pain	
REM sleep behaviour disorder	
Viral illnesses	
Wakefulness	

Cognitive symptoms	Sensory and perceptual symptoms
Confusion	Blurred vision
Changes in alertness	Hearing problems
False beliefs	Noise sensitivity
Fluctuating cognitive abilities	Poor visual perception of space
Lack of concentration	
Lack of decision-making abilities	
Lack of judgement	
Memory loss	
Reasoning problems	
Reduced attention span	

Motor symptoms	Behavioural and emotional symptoms
Loss of balance	Agitation
Rigid muscles	Distress
Shuffling walk	Frustration
Slowness of movement	Frightened
Slurred speech	Irritability
Shaky handwriting	Isolation
Tremor	Loss of enthusiasm
Trouble initiating movement	Mood changes
Unsteady gait	Nervousness
	Personality change
	Sudden outbursts
	Unpredictable nature
	Unresponsive behaviour

the progression of LBD. They are a significant source of distress to Thomas and can disturb his wife's sleep. Since developing LBD, Thomas has become sensitive to noise. People talking loudly or crowds of people talking can irritate him. However, he also cannot tolerate complete silence as he can "hear almost a complete buzzing in [his] brain".

Thomas experiences cognitive difficulties. On 6 October 2015, he underwent assessment on the Montreal Cognitive Assessment (MoCA). He scored 28/30, losing two points for delayed recall. The MoCA was repeated on 8 March 2016 and Thomas scored 29/30. The Addenbrooke's Cognitive Examination-Revised (ACE-R), which incorporates the Mini-Mental State Examination (MMSE), was conducted on 6 September 2017. Thomas scored 80/100 on ACE-R and 28/30 on MMSE (normal cognition). A score of 82/100 on ACE-R yields a 100% chance of having **dementia**. The domains on the ACE-R that were most problematic for Thomas were **memory** and **verbal fluency: attention** and orientation (18/18); memory (13/26); fluency (9/14); language (25/26); and visuospatial abilities (15/16) (see Figure 4.2). The visuospatial domain, an area of weakness in LBD,[18,19] was a relative strength for Thomas.

Thomas' wife reports some recent deterioration in his cognitive abilities. By way of illustration, she recounted difficulties he experienced while booking a trip to Australia in March 2020 for his daughter's wedding. Until this trip, Thomas had managed all online travel bookings without error. However, on this occasion he incorrectly booked their train journey to Dublin for the day before they intended to travel. Also, he booked the wrong hotel at the airport. Although both errors were rectified without serious consequence, they suggested to Thomas' wife that she could no longer leave him to complete such bookings unsupervised.

Thomas also exhibits significant psychiatric disturbances. He has experienced episodes of **depression** and **mania**. Thomas has written a book on his personal experience of LBD. His wife reports that during his "manic periods", he can write all day and night. On 20 July 2017, Thomas' doctor remarked in a letter to his neurologist that Thomas' behaviour can be volatile during the day, with the least thing upsetting him and causing him to become extremely agitated. That week, he had got out of the car while it was still moving, albeit slowly, after he had had an argument with his wife. Although Thomas had never been physical,

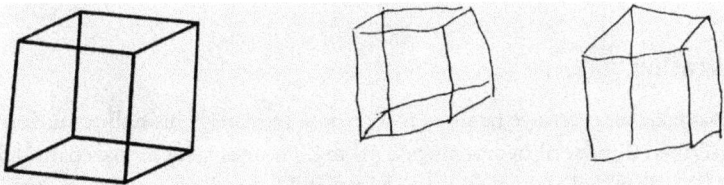

FIGURE 4.2 Thomas' drawing of the wire cube in visuospatial abilities in ACE-R (scored 1 of 2).

his wife had recently become afraid of him on account of his excessive agitation. In September 2017, Thomas was admitted to hospital following violent and threatening behaviour to his family and with confusion. His medical notes also show that he was suicidal in January 2018. He believed he had been visited by someone who told him he would be better off dead. However, he had no active suicide plan. In August 2018, Thomas had an impulsive suicide attempt following a fight with his son. His neurologist advised him to talk to his counsellor, whom he attended regularly, about the prospect of undertaking anger management.

Daily Activities

Thomas has always led a very full and active life. In 2006, he undertook a 10-day trek in South America for charity. He has been undaunted by challenges. In 2010, he emigrated to Australia with his wife. He was 45 years old at the time and most of his friends thought that this was too big a transition at this stage in his life. Prior to his diagnosis of LBD, Thomas had been a DJ and enjoyed miming to the music. Much of Thomas' earlier confidence and social interest has been compromised by LBD. He reports that he is afraid to be out late at night and hates being in large crowds or in a place that is very noisy or has loud music. Although Thomas concedes that LBD has had a profound impact on all aspects of his life, he has found it helpful to have structure to his days. He gets up around 8 a.m., has a cup of tea and toast and takes his medication. He then checks his phone and emails, contacts friends and speaks on social media with people with LBD from around the world. Thomas then sits or lies down and meditates using the Headspace app. He also does some light gardening or jobs in his workshop such as cutting up timber for the fire or making flower boxes.

   Thomas also tries to do some writing each day. He has written one book describing his personal journey with LBD and is currently working on a second book. When possible, Thomas goes for a drive with a friend. Once a week he visits his local pub to have a few drinks and meet friends. Other activities and interests he enjoys and finds helpful are doing jigsaws, being outside and listening to birds, keeping a couple of hens, collecting cattle with his friend, going to horse racing and watching sport on TV. Thomas is a strong advocate for people with LBD. He has participated in radio interviews and other activities designed to raise public awareness of LBD. He is also involved in a dementia working group.

Medication

Thomas takes an extensive range of medication. To manage his **hallucinations**, he is prescribed donepezil hydrochloride 10 mg. Thomas takes clonazepam 0.5 mg for REM sleep behaviour disorder. Most of Thomas' medication is unrelated to his LBD. For his gastro-intestinal problems, he takes Nexium 20 mg gastro-resistant tablets, lactulose fresenius 670 mg/ml oral solution and Movicol

13.8 g sachet, powder for oral solution. Thomas takes Amlode 10 mg tablets and Co-Diovan 160/12.5 mg tablets for high blood pressure. His asthma is treated using a salbutamol 100 mcg CFC-free inhaler and Flutiform 250/10 mcg. For pain management, Thomas is prescribed Durogesic DTrans 12 mcg per hour transdermal patches, OxyNorm 5 mg hard capsules and paracetamol 500 mg tablets. Finally, Thomas is prescribed diazepam Actavis 5 mg tablets as a muscle relaxant for his cervical **spinal stenosis**, especially when taking flights.

Communication

Thomas reports disruption to both his speech and writing as a result of LBD. He experiences slurred speech especially first thing in the morning: "it's like as if I am half drunk". He states that his speech will return to normal within about 15 minutes. He believes the size and clarity of his writing have also diminished. He describes how "as I write I go from big to small letters, very stretched out and from joined-up writing to printing". He also reports that he cannot even read his own writing after a couple of days. Thomas describes how he can sometimes stop mid-sentence in a conversation and must ask his interlocutor what they were talking about. This symptom "really torments and embarrasses" him. It can make him feel a little withdrawn and he admits that if he can get away without meeting people, he will do so.

Thomas was recorded in the morning of 10 March 2020. The recording was initially planned to take place in a hotel. However, because of the worsening Covid-19 situation, the interview and recording were conducted online instead. Thomas was on his own during the interview as his wife was meeting a friend prior to their trip to Australia for the wedding of Thomas' daughter. Thomas was alert and cooperative throughout the session. He was able to view all pictorial stimuli without difficulty and was not compromised in any way by the online mode of the interview. He found several of the tasks quite demanding, remarking at one point during the interview "phew, you're drawing all my resources today". However, even when tasks were particularly challenging, his response was good-natured and indicated a willingness to confront areas of difficulty. After the **letter fluency** task, he said, "that gave me almost a mental block … I'm delighted to have done that exercise actually".

Although Thomas reports slurring of his speech, especially when he wakes in the morning, his speech production was fully intelligible throughout the interview. There was no evidence of **dysarthria** or **apraxia of speech**. Thomas' **articulation** of speech sounds, breath control for speech, **resonance** and **voice quality** did not differ from these same speech parameters in adults without neurodegenerative disorder. Thomas used appropriate volume, stress and **intonation**. There was also no evidence of phonological impairment in Thomas' spoken output.

There is evidence of reduced speech rate and **fluency** in LBD. Speakers with LBD and **Parkinson's disease dementia** have been reported to have a speech rate of 73 words per minute.[20] This is considerably lower than the speech rate of 140 words per minute of 16 control speakers in the same study. However, Thomas' speech rate was 190 words per minute. This high speech rate is consistent with the speaking rate of Southern Irish speakers of English, the variety of English spoken by Thomas. In one study,[21] healthy male speakers of Southern Irish English had a speaking rate of 293 syllables per minute, a much higher speaking rate than is found in other varieties of English. Thomas had a speaking rate of 259 syllables per minute.

LBD speakers are also reported to have reduced speech fluency related to the increased duration of between-utterance pauses.[20] Thomas used pauses within and between utterances. They appeared to give him additional time in which to plan his utterances:

Within-utterance pause:

> they're mainly talking about like you said different countries as against what's going on in Australia which **(1.09)** gives me good hope

Between-utterance pause:

> I do suffer hallucinations am it's takin away the ability for me to drive **(2.0)** it's taken away an awful lot of my independence
> journeys in his jeep now would be just too rough **(2.59)** I'm not able to (1.29) you know I was go out to shed and cut a bit of timber and do little jobs like that and I can't do that anymore

A further source of dysfluency in Thomas' spoken output was his frequent phrase repetitions, particularly at the beginning of utterances. Like his use of pauses, these repetitions appeared to give Thomas additional time in which to plan his utterances:

> I think they I think they I think they ah (1.08) I don't think they took it serious
> I love the I love I love the ad [advocacy] we do a lot of advocacy work for the Alzheimer's Society

Thomas' morphological skills were intact. He was able to use a range of prefixes and inflectional and **derivational suffixes**:

Prefixes: <u>un</u>luckiest; <u>re</u>spray; <u>im</u>possibility
Inflectional suffixes: want<u>ed</u>; daughter<u>'s</u> wedding; sale<u>s</u>; young<u>est</u>
Derivational suffixes: passion<u>ate</u>; danger<u>ous</u>; construc<u>tion</u>; sick<u>ness</u>; self<u>ish</u>

Thomas displayed good comprehension of these same classes of morphemes when they were used by the investigator. He clearly understood the past participle *-ed* and plural *-s* **inflectional suffixes** in the investigator's first statement below, and the derivational suffixes *-ly* and *-ible* in the second statement below:

> you've really enjoy<u>ed</u> the job<u>s</u> you've work<u>ed</u> at
> think Lewy body is particular<u>ly</u> horr<u>ible</u>

Thomas also produced a range of complex grammatical constructions. In the first utterance below, he used a *that*-clause (underlined) which contained a **relative clause** (*which was a big deal*). In the second utterance, Thomas produced an **infinitive clause** (underlined) with a further infinitive clause (*to remember it*) embedded within it:

> I suppose <u>the high point of construction would be project manager of an apartment block in Five Dock in Sydney which was a big deal</u>
> I had <u>to draw on all my resources there to remember it</u>

However, Thomas also abandoned many grammatical constructions midstream. In the first utterance below, a relative clause is abandoned before the timed pause. Thomas abandons a **verb phrase** before the timed pause in the second utterance. These grammatical difficulties suggest a problem with the **planning** of utterances, with Thomas switching grammatical constructions midstream as he reworks the structure of his utterances:

> I ah was salesman for a wardrobe and shower screen company a small little company and it was a job that (1.52) I'd a life in Australia before I came home that you couldn't dream of
> I think it's more serious than people are, are (0.84) I don't think they're telling us everything

There was no evidence of impaired comprehension of **grammar**. Thomas was able to understand a wide range of grammatical constructions, including the embedded relative clauses (RC) in the first utterance (a comment) below and the interrogative **subordinate clause** (INT) in the second utterance (a question):

> you don't strike me as somebody [RC1 who sat in a job [RC2 that you didn't enjoy]]
> can you tell me a bit about [INT how Lewy body has affected your daily life]?

Thomas' lexical-semantic skills were also an area of strength. In the **confrontation naming** test, he named all items correctly apart from *French horn* which he called a *trombone* and then a *tuba*. Accurate naming was achieved following the presentation of an orthographic cue ('it begins with the letter F') and then a **phonemic cue**. There was no evidence during naming of visuo-perceptual errors or a category-specific deficit for living things, as has been demonstrated in previous research.[22,23] Thomas reported considerable struggle during the **category fluency** test. That said, his score of 16 animal names in 60 seconds significantly exceeded published category fluency scores for patients with LBD.[20,24,25] (It should be added that these studies involved older individuals than Thomas who were also in a more advanced state of cognitive decline.) Thomas' category fluency performance was lower than a score of 20.1 animal names in 60 seconds obtained by healthy participants aged 50–59 years.[26] This suggests that Thomas retained relatively efficient access to, and retrieval of words from, his mental lexicon. The slight decrement in his performance relative to healthy participants may be accounted for by some limitation of his executive control processes. This is supported by his **letter fluency** score of 11 words in 60 seconds. This score places Thomas above other individuals with LBD,[20,24] but behind healthy participants aged 50–59 years who produce on average 14 words in 60 seconds.[26] Thomas' letter and category fluency scores on ACE-R were 5/7 and 4/7, respectively.

In terms of sentence meaning, Thomas was able to use **subordinating conjunctions** to express a range of relations between actions and events. This included temporal and causal relations and the consequences of actions and states:

> my dad was a builder you see <u>so</u> I grew up (.) in construction
>
> (consequence)

> <u>because</u> she's doing the dishes (.) the sink is overflowing
>
> (causation)

> here we are 24 hours <u>before</u> we fly
>
> (time)

> <u>if</u> I enjoyed what I was doing I was good at it
>
> (condition)

> it's a dangerous place to be <u>because</u> I could see how you'd become isolated
>
> (reason)

Thomas was also able to represent several participant or **semantic roles** in the utterances he produced. They included **agent**, theme, source, location, patient and beneficiary:

> the young fella[AGENT] is takin (2.61) cookies[THEME] out of the jar[SOURCE]

we[AGENT] all sat around the table[LOCATION] up on a deck[LOCATION]
we[AGENT] do a lot of advocacy work[PATIENT] for the Alzheimer's
Society[BENEFICIARY]

Thomas displayed strengths and weaknesses in the **pragmatics** of language. He
was adept at using **figurative language** including **idiom**, **metaphor**, proverb
and **hyperbole**:

my life is literally an open book

(idiom)

I was at the height of my career

(metaphor)

The apple does not fall far from the tree

(proverb)

I wash my hands ten (.) a hundred times a day

(hyperbole)

Thomas also had intact comprehension of non-literal language used by the
author, including in the expressions *rising from the ashes*, *taking a toll on one's
health* and *keeping one's fingers crossed*. Other pragmatic skills included Thomas'
use of self-initiated self-repair to correct information, hedges to acknowledge a
topic digression, **presupposition** to represent mutual background knowledge,
and **deixis** to relate utterances to spatial, temporal and other aspects of context.
Thomas also made skilled use of verbal **humour**:

Self-initiated self-repair:

the reason I put <u>two reasons I put</u> it off one was I was pretty ill since
Christmas

Hedge:

I don't stress except for this coronavirus but <u>that's another, another story</u>

Presupposition:

<u>it was</u> stress that led me to my first (.) health problems (cleft construction)
→ something led to the first health problems

Deixis:

there's two and a half thousand people living <u>here</u>

(spatial deixis)

Humour:

> I know people have when they have to hear it from someone else to believe that you're actually as bad you say I think, I think it might be an Irish thing I think that that's why so many go to funerals to make sure they're dead (*laughter*)

Thomas was able to switch between the idiomatic and literal meanings of words as illustrated in the following exchange. In Thomas' first utterance, the word *book* is part of an idiomatic expression *open book*. The author then uses the **pronoun** *it* to refer to the book on LBD that Thomas has written. This requires that Thomas switch to the literal meaning of *book* which he was clearly able to do:

THO: there's nothing you can't ask me my life is literally an open book
INV: well I got it
THO: ah thank you
INV: and I've been wanting to get you to sign it but that's for another day

Thomas was able to tailor his utterances in accordance with his interlocutor's knowledge. This is illustrated in the utterance below where Thomas is seen to rework his utterance to accommodate the hearer's state of knowledge. Thomas sets out to say that he loves his advocacy work. However, he then realises that the author does not know that he undertakes advocacy work for the Alzheimer's Society and must be told this first, before going on to say that he loves this work:

> I love the I love I love the ad [advocacy] we do a lot of advocacy work for the Alzheimer's Society which I, I love that

The ability to tailor utterances to the knowledge or, in this case, lack of knowledge of a hearer is an important pragmatic language skill that depends on **theory of mind** (ToM), the cognitive capacity to attribute mental states to one's own and others' minds. Cognitive decline in LBD is associated with reduced recognition of facial expressions associated with the **affective mental states** of sadness, fear, anger, surprise and disgust.[27] However, as well as being able to attribute mental states to his interlocutor in conversation, Thomas also attributed mental states to the characters in the Cookie Theft picture. He described how the children in the picture *knew* that the mother was *distracted*. This is second-order ToM reasoning, namely, the attribution to the children of a mental state (knowledge) about another person's mental state (the mother's state of distraction). Thomas was also able to attribute mental states to the mind of the young girl in the picture. She was gesturing to her brother to be quiet. This **gesture** only made sense to the extent that the girl entertained a specific mental state, namely, the *desire* to avoid detection by their mother:

they know that their mother is distracted
the young lady is telling him to be quiet, so she won't be heard

On other occasions, Thomas was imperceptive to the intentions and mental states of characters in a picture. In his narration of the Flowerpot Incident, Thomas could not establish a key mental state of the man in the picture who was struck on the head by a falling flowerpot. Although acknowledging that the man was upset and angry ("he starts giving out about it"), he was unable to work out that the man enters the building and bangs on the woman's door because he *wants* to remonstrate with her over the incident. This mental state or intention is never identified by Thomas, as his comments at the end of the narrative reveal:

> I just can't make sense of we'll say the top the top picture where he goes in the door and why is he banging the door down here (1.45) it just doesn't make sense to me

Occasionally, Thomas made remarks in conversation the relevance of which was not immediately apparent to his interlocutor. In the following exchange, the author has just asked Thomas if he has any favourite TV programmes. Thomas initially responds by saying that he has. However, at T3 and T5, he remarks that LBD is worst at night, before going on to name some of the programmes he enjoys watching in T7 and T9. The author must attempt to establish the relevance of these remarks. One possible relevance is that because Thomas' LBD is worst at night, this is when he watches most TV if he cannot sleep. While this is a plausible **inference** for the hearer to draw, Thomas has clearly failed to fulfil a conversational expectation to make manifest the relevance of his utterances:

T1: THO: I, I have
T2: INV: um hum
→ **T3: THO:** am (1.52) one thing about Lewy body dementia
T4: INV: um
→ **T5: THO:** it's at night (1.00) that it really comes into play
T6: INV: um
T7: THO: comedies like *The Big Bang Theory*
T8: INV: right
T9: THO: *Friends, Fawlty Towers, Fools and Horses*
T10: INV: yeah, yeah
T11: THO: absolutely love them

Like pragmatics, Thomas displayed both strengths and weaknesses in his use of **discourse**. He made skilled use of **cohesive devices** to link utterances in discourse, including **ellipsis**, **anaphoric reference** and **lexical substitution**:

Ellipsis:

> if I enjoyed what I was doing, I was good at it (.) you know and if I
> didn't enjoy it (0.81) I wasn't [*good at it*]

Anaphoric reference:

> they held <u>two rounds of dementia awareness evenings all over the country</u>
> and I absolutely loved doing <u>that</u>
> [*wife's name*] has spent time in (.) <u>Chengdu in China</u> (.) doing reflexology
> I spent two weeks <u>there</u>

Lexical substitution:

> it's probably the wrong thing to say but if I had a choice of dementias ah,
> ah I wouldn't pick this <u>one</u>

Thomas was also able to use complex forms of discourse. In the following
exchange, the main discourse is suspended temporarily at T3 and T5 to allow
Thomas to explain his remark that there are times that he is "not up to writing".
Thomas is using meta-discourse in these turns before returning to the main
discourse:

T1: THO: If I'm, if I'm here in the afternoon and (1.30) if I'm not up to writing
T2: INV: um
T3: THO: and there's times I can't write because you just
T4: INV: um
T5: THO: it won't come to you
T6: INV: um hum
T7: THO: I love watching shows like the, *The Chase*

Thomas also made use of **direct reported speech**, a form of discourse that requires
a complex interplay between cognitive, linguistic and pragmatic skills: [28]

> there's nights I would think that I'd be after havin' a good night's sleep
> and [*wife's name*] would say to me "God, you'd a bad night last night"

Against these discourse strengths, Thomas tended to omit information from discourse. This occurred during the Sam and Fred story, where his recall of information was dependent on **memory**. Although Thomas was able to recall the gist
of the story, he omitted details such as that the crops were washed away by the
storm, the storm ripped open the barn door and temporal information, including
the number of years the brothers had farmed together and the time of day when
the animals were returned to the barn:

Sam and Fred story (immediate recall):

> so, Sam and Fred, Sam and Fred, Sam and Fred, so the best the best I can give you about that is that they were farmers (.) ahhh they watched the weather ahhh they had an idea what was coming (3.17) the weather was worse than they thought aammm (3.52) was sheep and cattle or was it sheep and pigs I'm not sure (.) but animals broke free and (.) was it neighbours or people in the village (.) helped them to round up that's as much as I could

Thomas' Cinderella story also lacked detail. There was no mention of the mal-treatment that Cinderella suffered, that she had two stepsisters, that the fairy godmother cast a spell that required Cinderella to leave the ball by midnight, that Cinderella danced with the prince at the ball, and that a royal courtier tried the slipper on the feet of women who had attended the ball. On only one occasion did Thomas identify when he had omitted information and moved to correct it. This occurred towards the end of the narrative. Thomas rather precipitously concluded the story by saying that Cinderella and the prince got married only to rework his ending to include the fitting of the shoe:

Cinderella:

> her friends the mice got the key and (.) they let her out and they got married (.) the shoe fit the shoe ah the shoe fit desh [xxx (*unintelligible*)] the slipper that was lost obviously fitted her they got married

Thomas displayed some information-sequencing problems. He stated for the first time that Cinderella must leave the ball by midnight *after* she spent the evening dancing with the prince, even though it was an important part of the fairy god-mother's magic spell. Thomas' problems with the ordering of information were relatively minor compared to his difficulties with the omission of information.

COMMUNICATION PROFILE:

Speech intelligibility:

- Thomas displayed fully intelligible speech production; there was no motor speech disorder or evidence of phonological impairment; his speech rate was elevated relative to both healthy individuals and people with LBD but was consistent with the speaking rate of speakers of Southern Irish English; multiple phrase repetitions particularly at the beginning of utterances compromised fluency.

Morphology and syntax:

- Thomas used and understood a range of inflectional and derivational morphemes; he was able to produce and understand complex syntax; Thomas abandoned many grammatical constructions midstream.

Vocabulary and semantics:

- Thomas displayed strong lexical-semantic skills; he produced only one error during confrontation naming and there was no evidence of lexical, semantic or visuo-perceptual errors in other contexts; some mild word-finding difficulty may be present in conversation; Thomas expressed complex conceptual relations in sentences and used a range of semantic roles to represent entities and participants.

Pragmatics:

- Thomas displayed strengths in several areas of pragmatics: figurative language, conversational repair, hedges, presupposition, deixis and humour; he could switch between idiomatic and literal meaning and tailor utterances to his hearer's knowledge; he could attribute mental states to characters but struggled on occasion to establish intentions; the relevance of some utterances was not made manifest.

Discourse:

- Thomas was adept at using cohesive devices to link utterances in various types of discourse; he also used complex discourse such as meta-discourse and direct reported speech; he tended to capture the gist of narratives while omitting detailed information; there were occasional difficulties with the sequencing of events in discourse.

Cognition:

- Lengthy pauses between and within utterances suggested Thomas needed additional time in which to plan his utterances; that executive control processes were an area of difficulty was also indicated by Thomas' reduced phonemic and category fluency scores relative to healthy individuals (but not individuals with LBD); Thomas was assessed on the MoCA and ACE-R, with memory and verbal fluency most impaired; Thomas displayed first- and second-order theory of mind skills, although he struggled to establish intentions of actors in some contexts.

Suggestions for Further Reading

(1) Walker, Z., Possin, K.L., Boeve, B.F. and Aarsland, D. (2015) 'Non-Alzheimer's dementia 2: Lewy body dementias', *Lancet*, 386 (10004): 1683–1697.

This article provides a comprehensive overview of LBD. It examines the epidemiology, pathogenesis, genetics, diagnosis and clinical symptoms of LBD. Other issues addressed include neuropsychological aspects and management. The discussion serves as a useful medical primer for readers in speech-language pathology with little prior knowledge of LBD.

(2) Gross, R.G., Camp, E., McMillan, C.T., Dreyfuss, M., Gunawardena, D., Cook, P.A., Morgan, B., Siderowf, A., Hurtig, H.I., Stern, M.B. and Grossman, M. (2013) 'Impairment of script comprehension in Lewy body spectrum disorders', *Brain and Language*, 125 (3): 330–343.

This article is one of the few studies to examine higher-order language comprehension in LBD. The investigators examined the ability of healthy seniors and individuals with Parkinson's disease and Parkinson's disease dementia (PDD)/LBD to judge the order of events in a script. Impairment of this ability in participants with PDD/LBD was related to executive dysfunction. This receptive deficit mirrors the results of earlier studies, which found an expressive deficit in event ordering during narrative production that was also related to executive dysfunction but was unrelated to lexical semantics and grammar.[29,30]

(3) Grossman, M., Gross, R.G., Moore, P., Dreyfuss, M., McMillan, C.T., Cook, P.A., Ash, S. and Siderowf, A. (2011) 'Difficulty processing temporary syntactic ambiguities in Lewy body spectrum disorder', *Brain and Language,* 120 (1): 52–60.

This paper demonstrates that impairments of executive control are not only involved in narrative comprehension and production problems in LBD. The authors found that slowed processing of sentences with structural ambiguities, half of which had been lengthened between the onset of the ambiguity and its resolution, was related to working memory deficits in individuals with PDD/LBD.

Questions

(1) Thomas made extensive use of figurative language in conversation including *metaphor, proverb* and *hyperbole*. Identify what type of figurative language is used in each of the following utterances:

(a) "it was just a roller coaster from there to where I am today"
(b) "I'm probably be the most unluckiest man on the planet"
(c) "I suppose the high point of construction would be project manager of an apartment block"

    (d) "when you push the boat out too far you can't get back"
    (e) "it might take you off the road you're on but there is another road there and not give up"

(2) Thomas was adept at using cohesive devices to link his utterances in discourse. This included *lexical substitution, ellipsis* and *anaphoric reference*. What type of cohesion is Thomas using in the following utterances?

    (a) "I like being on my own but I'm afraid of it"
    (b) **INV:** do you have a favourite TV programme or maybe a few favourites? THO: I have
    (c) "that's what holidays are I, I, I'm like this one unfortunately we're going tomorrow night"
    (d) **INV:** do you recall the Cinderella story it's probably not? THO: I do
    (e) "the job moves him around the country he's never in the one place too long and he just loves it"

(3) Thomas tended to omit information and occasionally presented information in the wrong order. However, he was able to rework his utterances to provide his hearer with more *specific information* and with *background information* when that was needed to understand what he was saying. Thomas also explicitly *rejected information* when he realised that it might be inferred from something he said. Which of these uses of information in italics applies to the utterances below?

    (a) "because a doctor, a German doctor in Australia advised me to give up construction"
    (b) "I can't swim but I'd go into the water for twenty minutes"
    (c) "everyone knows me because I have been on, because of the book I've been on radio I've been on television I've been on the newspapers and everyone knows what I have"
    (d) "I'm not a very religious guy but [wife's name] would be up maybe at six (.) and I might get up an I'd go to the local church"
    (e) "I have an interest in the horses I'm not a big gambler but there's two guys that take me racing and say I pick a horse number nine"

Answers

(1) (a) metaphor
    (b) hyperbole
    (c) metaphor
    (d) proverb
    (e) metaphor
(2) (a) anaphoric reference
    (b) ellipsis
    (c) lexical substitution

    (d) ellipsis

    (e) anaphoric reference

(3) (a) specific information: a doctor is revised to become a German doctor.

    (b) reject information: Thomas explicitly states that he cannot swim as he realises his hearer might infer that he can swim when he says he goes into the water for 20 minutes.

    (c) background information: Thomas is about to say he has been on radio but then reworks his utterance to say that it is because he has written a book that he has been on radio and everyone knows that he has LBD.

    (d) reject information: Thomas explicitly states that he is not religious as he realises his hearer might infer that he is religious when he says he attends the local church.

    (e) reject information: Thomas explicitly states that he is not a big gambler as he realises his hearer might infer that he is a big gambler when he says he has an interest in horses and goes to the races.

References

[1] Kane, J.P., Surendranathan, A., Bentley, A., Barker, S.A.H., Taylor, J.P., Thomas, A.J., Allan, L.M., McNally, R.J., James, P.W., McKeith, I.G., Burn, D.J. and O'Brien, J.T. (2018) 'Clinical prevalence of Lewy body dementia', *Alzheimer's Research & Therapy*, 10 (1): 19. doi: 1186/s13195-018-0350-6.

[2] Zaccai, J., McCracken, C. and Brayne, C. (2005) 'A systematic review of prevalence and incidence studies of dementia with Lewy bodies', *Age and Ageing*, 34 (6): 561–566.

[3] Savica, R., Grossardt, B.R., Bower, J.H., Boeve, B.F., Ahlskog, J.E. and Rocca, W.A. (2013) 'Incidence of dementia with Lewy bodies and Parkinson's disease dementia', *JAMA Neurology*, 70 (11): 1396–1402.

[4] Yang, S.K., Chen, W., Su, C.H. and Liu, C.H. (2018) 'Incidence and comorbidity of dementia with Lewy bodies: A population-based cohort study', *Behavioural Neurology*, 2018: 7631951. doi: 1155/2018/7631951.

[5] Moutin, A., Blanc, F., Gros, A., Manera, V., Fabre, R., Sauleau, E., Gomez-Luporsi, I., Tifratene, K., Friedman, L., Thümmler, S., Pradier, C., Robert, P.H. and David, R. (2018) 'Sex ratio in dementia with Lewy bodies balanced between Alzheimer's disease and Parkinson's disease dementia: A cross-sectional study', *Alzheimer's Research & Therapy*, 10 (1): 92. doi: 10.1186/s13195-018-0417-4.

[6] Boot, B.P., Orr, C.F., Ahlskog, J.E., Ferman, T.J., Roberts, R., Pankratz, V.S., Dickson, D.W., Parisi, J., Aakre, J.A., Geda, Y.E., Knopman, D.S., Petersen, R.C. and Boeve, B.F. (2013) 'Risk factors for dementia with Lewy bodies', *Neurology*, 81 (9): 833–840.

[7] Eversfield, C.L. and Orton, L.D. (2019) 'Auditory and visual hallucination prevalence in Parkinson's disease and dementia with Lewy bodies: A systematic review and meta-analysis', *Psychological Medicine*, 49 (14): 2342–2353.

[8] Tsunoda, N., Hashimoto, M., Ishikawa, T., Fukuhara, R., Yuki, S., Tanaka, H., Hatada, Y., Miyagawa, Y. and Ikeda, M. (2018) 'Clinical features of auditory hallucinations in patients with dementia with Lewy bodies: A soundtrack of visual hallucinations', *Journal of Clinical Psychiatry*, 79 (3): pii. doi: 10.4088/JCP.17m11623.

[9] Nagahama, Y., Okina, T., Suzuki, N., Matsuda, M., Fukao, K. and Murai, T. (2007) 'Classification of psychotic symptoms in dementia with Lewy bodies', *American Journal of Geriatric Psychiatry*, 15 (11): 961–967.

[10] Shea, Y.F., Ha, J. and Chu, L.-W. (2015) 'Comparisons of clinical symptoms in bio-marker-confirmed Alzheimer's disease, dementia with Lewy bodies, and frontotemporal dementia patients in a local memory clinic', *Psychogeriatrics*, 15 (4): 235–241.

[11] Tzeng, R.C., Tsai, C.F., Wang, C.T., Wang, T.Y. and Chiu, P.Y. (2018) 'Delusions in patients with dementia with Lewy bodies and the associated factors', *Behavioural Neurology*, 2018 (2018): 6707291. doi: 10.1155/2018/6707291.

[12] Yoo, H.S., Jeon, S., Chung, S.J., Yun, M., Lee, P.H., Sohn, Y.H., Evans, A.C. and Ye, B.S. (2018) 'Olfactory dysfunction in Alzheimer's disease- and Lewy body-related cognitive impairment', *Alzheimer's & Dementia*, 14 (10): 1243–1252.

[13] Beagle, A.J., Darwish, S.M., Ranasinghe, K.G., La, A.L., Karageorgiou, E. and Vossel, K.A. (2017) 'Relative incidence of seizures and myoclonus in Alzheimer's disease, dementia with Lewy bodies, and frontotemporal dementia', *Journal of Alzheimer's Disease*, 60 (1): 211–223.

[14] Mueller, C., Soysal, P., Rongve, A., Isik, A.T., Thompson, T., Maggi, S., Smith, L. Basso, C., Stewart, R., Ballard, C., O'Brien, J.T., Aarsland, D., Stubbs, B. and Veronese, N. (2019) 'Survival time and differences between dementia with Lewy bodies and Alzheimer's disease following diagnosis: A meta-analysis of longitudinal studies', *Ageing Research Reviews*, 50: 72–80.

[15] Fereshtehnejad, S.M., Lökk, J., Wimo, A. and Eriksdotter, M. (2018) 'No significant difference in cognitive decline and mortality between Parkinson's disease dementia and dementia with Lewy bodies: Naturalistic longitudinal data from the Swedish Dementia Registry', *Journal of Parkinson's Disease*, 8 (4): 553–561.

[16] Price, A., Farooq, R., Yuan, J.M., Menon, V.B., Cardinal, R.N. and O'Brien, J.T. (2017) 'Mortality in dementia with Lewy bodies compared with Alzheimer's dementia: A retrospective naturalistic cohort study', *BMJ Open*, 7 (11): e017504. doi: 10.1136/bmjopen-2017-017504.

[17] Armstrong, M.J., Alliance, S., Corsentino, P., DeKosky, S.T. and Taylor, A. (2019) 'Cause of death and end-of-life experiences in individuals with dementia with Lewy bodies', *Journal of the American Geriatrics Society*, 67 (1): 67–73.

[18] Johnson, D.K., Morris, J.C. and Galvin, J.E. (2005) 'Verbal and visuospatial deficits in dementia with Lewy bodies', *Neurology*, 65 (8): 1232–1238.

[19] Hamilton, J.M., Salmon, D.P., Galasko, D., Raman, R., Emond, J., Hansen, L.A., Masliah, E. and Thal, L.J. (2008) 'Visuospatial deficits predict rate of cognitive decline in autopsy-verified dementia with Lewy bodies', *Neuropsychology*, 22 (6): 729–737.

[20] Ash, S., McMillan, C., Gross, R.G., Cook, P., Gunawardena, D., Morgan, B., Boller, A., Siderowf, A. and Grossman, M. (2012) 'Impairments of speech fluency in Lewy body spectrum disorder', *Brain and Language*, 120 (3): 290–302.

[21] Lee, A. and Doherty, R. (2017) 'Speaking rate and articulation rate of native speakers of Irish English', *Speech, Language and Hearing*, 20 (4): 206–211.

[22] Williams, V.G., Bruce, J.M., Westervelt, H.J., Davis, J.D., Grace, J., Malloy, P.F. and Tremont, G. (2007) 'Boston naming performance distinguishes between Lewy body and Alzheimer's dementias', *Archives of Clinical Neuropsychology*, 22 (8): 925–931.

[23] Laws, K.R., Crawford, J.R., Gnoato, F. and Sartori, G. (2007) 'A preponderance of category deficits for living things in Alzheimer's disease and Lewy body dementia', *Journal of the International Neuropsychological Society*, 13 (3): 401–409.

[24] Gnanalingham, K.K., Byrne, E.J., Thornton, A., Sambrook, M.A. and Bannister, P. (1997) 'Motor and cognitive function in Lewy body dementia: Comparison with Alzheimer's and Parkinson's diseases', *Journal of Neurology, Neurosurgery, and Psychiatry*, 62 (3): 243–252.

[25] Nagahama, Y., Okina, T. and Suzuki, N. (2017) 'Neuropsychological differences related to age in dementia with Lewy bodies', *Dementia and Geriatric Cognitive Disorders Extra*, 7 (2): 188–194.

[26] Tombaugh, T.N., Kozakb, J. and Reesc, L. (1999) 'Normative data stratified by age and education for two measures of verbal fluency: FAS and animal naming', *Archives of Clinical Neuropsychology*, 14 (2): 167–177.

[27] Kojma, Y., Kumagai, T., Hidaka, T., Kakamu, T., Endo, S., Mori, Y., Tsukamoto, T., Sakamoto, T., Murata, M., Hayakawa, T. and Fukushima, T. (2018) 'Characteristics of facial expression recognition ability in patients with Lewy body disease', *Environmental Health and Preventive Medicine*, 23 (1): 32. doi: 10.1186/s12199=018-0723-2.

[28] Cummings, L. (2016) 'Reported speech: A clinical pragmatic perspective', in A. Capone, F. Kiefer & F. Lo Piparo (eds), *Indirect Reports and Pragmatics*, Series: Perspectives in Pragmatics, Philosophy & Psychology, Vol. 5, Cham, Switzerland: Springer International Publishing AG, 31–55.

[29] Ash, S., McMillan, C., Gross, R.G., Cook, P., Morgan, B., Boller, A., Dreyfuss, M., Siderowf, A. and Grossman, M. (2011) 'The organization of narrative discourse in Lewy body spectrum disorder', *Brain and Language*, 119 (1): 30–41.

[30] Ash, S., Xie, S.X., Gross, R.G., Dreyfuss, M., Boller, A., Camp, E., Morgan, B., O'Shea, J. and Grossman, M. (2012) 'The organization and anatomy of narrative comprehension and expression in Lewy body spectrum disorders', *Neuropsychology*, 26 (3): 368–384.

CASE STUDY 5

Multiple Sclerosis

KEY FACTS AND FIGURES

- Multiple sclerosis (MS) is an autoimmune disease of the central nervous system (CNS) that is characterised by focal inflammation, demyelination and axonal injury. It is the most common inflammatory neurological disease in young adults, affecting some 2,221,188 people globally in 2016.[1]
- MS prevalence varies significantly with geographical region. There is a high prevalence in North America and Europe and a low prevalence in Eastern Asia and sub-Saharan Africa. In the United States, the estimated 2010 prevalence of MS cumulated over 10 years was 309.2 per 100,000.[2] Prevalence was higher in women than in men (female: male ratio of 2.8) and in the 55- to 64-year age group than other age groups. A US north–south decreasing prevalence gradient was identified. In 2006, the prevalence of MS was 13.1 per 100,000 in Tokachi province, Japan.[3]
- Environmental predictors of MS risk include vitamin D status, obesity in early life, infection with the Epstein-Barr virus and cigarette smoking.[4] MS is partially heritable, with genes that affect the immune response contributing to heritability.
- There are currently four MS phenotypes: relapsing-remitting MS; clinically isolated syndrome; primary progressive MS; and secondary progressive MS. Life expectancy is influenced by MS phenotype.[5] Relapse phenotype (cerebellar, pyramidal, bowel/bladder) is associated with disability outcomes.[6]

DOI: 10.4324/9781003153559-6

- MS is associated with motor and sensory problems, cognitive difficulties, speech and swallowing disorders, and psychiatric issues. Dysarthria and dysphagia affect approximately 40% and 38% of patients with MS, respectively.[7,8] Cognitive impairments occur in 45–65% of people with MS.[9,10] In 200 younger patients with MS, fatigue (61%) was the most commonly reported symptom, with six other symptoms with a prevalence greater than 50%: visual disturbances; impaired mobility; dizziness; pain; spasticity; and sleep disorders.[11] Fatigue (77.4%), numbness/tingling (70.0%) and walking or balance problems (68.8%) were the most common symptoms experienced in MS relapse in 5,311 patients.[12] Communication and swallowing problems in MS have a significant negative impact on quality of life.[13]

Background

Samantha (not her real name) is 50;5 years old. She is married and is mother to three boys aged 7, 19 and 21 years. She was diagnosed with MS in March 2007. However, she had unexplained symptoms for many years prior to her diagnosis. In 1987 and 1988, she experienced right facial paralysis which affected her speech and ability to drink. Several tests were performed at two hospitals. Doctors diagnosed her with borderline MS, although she was unaware of this diagnosis at the time. In 2002, she experienced tingling sensations and pins and needles in her right leg. She had a further episode of right facial paralysis in 2006. Samantha's family doctor attributed many of these symptoms to stress. In October 2006, Samantha developed blurry vision and then had no vision in her right eye. She reported that she was exhausted at this time and had low mood. She attended the accident and emergency department of her local area hospital and was referred to the eye clinic at a large regional hospital. She received onward referral to the neurology department where she underwent several tests. In December 2006, she had an MRI scan. It was these investigations that led to a definitive diagnosis of MS in March 2007. Samantha's sister and first cousin also have MS. She is a university graduate.

Samantha had her youngest son after her MS diagnosis. The pregnancy and delivery were normal, and she experienced a period of good health following the birth. Samantha no longer works. Before leaving employment in August 2016, she worked as a corporate and trust fund raiser for a charity. She described this role as "hard work" and "quite stressful" but also very rewarding: "it was really good to see money coming in and to see older people getting value out of it". Samantha has continued to pursue many different activities since her diagnosis. In 2007, she went to Tanzania for 16 days with The Leprosy Mission and took part in a house construction project. She worked as an assistant in the kitchen and was also involved in the construction work. Her neurologist was concerned that she would find the conditions very difficult (temperatures were 40+ degrees), but she experienced good health while she was there and described her time in Tanzania as "amazing". Samantha enjoys walking, making jam and reading, although her pleasure in reading has been reduced on account of her vision problems. She is involved in various church activities and assists with pastoral work. Samantha attends a weekly MS exercise class under the auspices of the MS Society in her local leisure centre. This has social as well as physical benefits for her. She watches TV and particularly enjoys programmes like *Escape to the Country*.

Clinical Symptoms

Samantha has experienced a wide range of symptoms as a result of her MS. Her balance and **coordination** are affected. She can walk unaided but reports that when she walks with someone, she constantly bumps into them. Samantha has been given exercises by the neuro-physiotherapist to improve her balance and coordination. The physiotherapist also told her that while her mobility is good, there is a need to strengthen her core. Since August 2019, when Samantha's neurologist believes she had a relapse, she has experienced abnormal sensation in her right leg. This followed a 200-mile round car trip to visit her mother who had been in hospital. The numbness in her right leg and foot were such that she needed to use Nordic poles to walk. She also had to stop driving as she was unable to use the brake in her car. In November 2019, her neurologist requested that another MRI scan be undertaken. This was to establish if her symptoms were caused by a new lesion or a reactivated old lesion.

Samantha's vision has deteriorated. She uses glasses now all the time for reading, otherwise written text appears blurred. Memory is often impaired in MS, with deficits reported in **short-term memory, working memory** and long-term memory.[14,15] Samantha reports that her memory is poor and that she cannot hold thoughts in her head for any length of time. When she reads, she cannot remember what she has read a short time later. She often forgets what she was saying in conversation and what a conversation is about. She has never had a formal cognitive assessment. Samantha experiences problems with bladder control and has appointments with the continence nurse. She has persistent fatigue that has not been alleviated by medication. On some days, her fatigue is so severe that she is unable to get out of bed. In October 2018, Samantha visited a nutritionist and was given dietary advice (e.g. reduce coffee intake). This resulted in a reduction of her fatigue. Samantha experiences low mood and mild **depression**. Depression is common in MS, with a lifetime **prevalence** of approximately 50%.[16]

Daily Activities

MS has had a negative impact on everything that Samantha does in her life. She reports having no enthusiasm for daily activities and that while tasks are still done, she undertakes them more slowly than usual. Samantha can do the laundry, ironing, shopping and cooking. Leisure and social activities have been adversely affected by MS. She still tries to go for walks, weather permitting. MS severely affected Samantha's occupational functioning when she was in employment. When she experienced relapses and symptoms, she had to take extended periods of time off work. In 2007 and 2008, she was permitted to work from home. All daily activities are compromised by fatigue. There are days when she is unable to take her youngest son to school because she is so debilitated by fatigue.

Medication

In October 2012, Samantha was prescribed amantadine and modafinal to treat fatigue. However, she did not find these drugs effective, and stopped taking them. She takes no other medication related to her MS.

Communication

Samantha reports several communication difficulties related to her MS. She can say something, and then realises that what she thought she had said is not what she did in fact say. She often gets the names of things wrong. She can "blurt out" statements randomly in conversation and constantly feels "all over the place" during conversation. She believes her communication difficulties have contributed to a reduction in her confidence and made it more difficult for her to maintain her social network. The restrictions in social participation described by Samantha are commonly reported in people with MS.[17] Samantha also thinks the absence of employment may be contributing to her communication problems, in that she is not required to make the same extensive use of her communication skills at home as she did in the workplace.

The author visited Samantha at home on the morning of 13 August 2018. She was at home by herself. We worked at a table in her kitchen. Samantha was keen to communicate and chatted at length as she prepared coffee before the recording commenced. She had a warm rapport and was an able, enthusiastic communicator. She followed all task instructions with ease and clarified points when necessary (e.g. she asked if the six pictures in the Flowerpot Incident task were all part of a single story). Samantha appeared not to fatigue during the session but reported considerable fatigue after the visit.

When **dysarthria** arises in MS, it is typically ataxic-spastic and affects several speech production sub-systems.[18] However, Samantha's speech production skills were intact and there was no evidence of dysarthria or **apraxia of speech**. Her

articulation of speech sounds, breath control for speech, **voice quality** and use of **resonance** were similar to these same speech parameters in adults without neurodegenerative disorder. Samantha's volume, stress and **intonation**, speech rate and **fluency** were also within the normal range. Speakers with MS have been found to have extended pause times between responses, a behaviour that may be related either to speech difficulties or to slowed information processing.[19] Pause duration and frequency in MS also increase with the cognitive load of a speech task.[20] Samantha often had lengthy filled and unfilled pauses between a task instruction and her production of a response. For example, when asked to put the word *tree* into a sentence, she uttered "(2:77) emmmm (.) I have a view which is of lots of trees". There was no evidence of phonological impairment in Samantha's speech.

Samantha's utterances were well-formed for the most part. She displayed intact use of inflectional and **derivational morphology**, and expressed a range of **clauses** in her utterances:

Inflectional morphology:

younger; relapses; welcomes; wearing; realised; Jack's favourite

Derivational morphology:

requirements; location; adviser; relatively; dreadful; dangerous; disappear; princess

Clauses:

I don't know [how I did it]

(*interrogative*)

knowing that there was going to be a turn in the weather em which happened a lot quicker [than they were expecting]

(*comparative*)

I would have went in [to promote self-employment]

(*infinitive*)*

it's not the estate agent but the person [who's showing them round]

(*relative*)

*[*Note*: 'have went' is a grammatical feature of Samantha's **dialect**, Northern Irish English]

When problems with **syntax** did arise in Samantha's expressive language, they appeared to be related to her cognitive difficulties. Quite often, she simply abandoned utterances midway as if she had lost track of what she was intending to say. This is consistent with her self-reported problems with **memory** which meant that she often forgot what she was intending to say in conversation. In each of the following examples, Samantha abandons an utterance at the point indicated by ↑:

I was in the kitchen as opposed to me, me ↑ I remember the neurologist
…

I came home and I had so many stories but that, that was great yes, I've had
↑ but you know …

I don't inject myself or any of that there am (.) so it didn't ↑ but of late it
really has impacted on me

Samantha was also able to comprehend utterances that contained complex syntax. She had no difficulty understanding the interrogative ($_{INT}$) and relative ($_{REL}$) **subordinate clauses** embedded in the following questions posed by the author:

Can you tell me [$_{INT}$ what you were doing before you left the workplace]?

Can you tell me about a holiday [$_{REL}$ that you've taken]?

When sentence comprehension difficulties arise in MS, they are often associated with compromised information-processing speed.[21] Given that Samantha appeared to need more time to plan sentence production, slowed information processing may also play a part in her sentence comprehension, even as she is able to comprehend utterances with complex syntax.

People with MS are reported to produce naming errors during testing. Visual errors suggestive of perceptual deficits, superordinate responses and phonological deficits are among the errors that speakers with MS produce.[22,23] Errors arise when semantic, visual and rhyming cues are used to elicit target words.[24] Samantha's lexical-semantic skills were an area of relative strength. There were only two pictures that she struggled to identify during the **confrontation naming** task. On both occasions, her incorrect responses were semantically related to the target word. The word 'lobster' was initially named as *prawn*. However, following a **semantic cue** ("it is something a bit bigger than a prawn"), Samantha replied "it's not a lobster". Samantha produced *mermaid* and *sea urchin* for 'seahorse' before saying "it's a horse something horse". There was no evidence that Samantha experienced a **word-finding difficulty** in conversation. Although she made extensive use of the **filler** *em* (6.2 instances per minute), the location of this particle – at syntactic boundaries and *not* before **content words** – suggests that its presence may be related more to the syntactic **planning** and encoding of utterances (and the need for more time for this planning and encoding) than to **lexical retrieval**:

the sink is overflowing and <u>em</u> she has water (.) sort of spilling down onto the floor

it was after I got diagnosed with the MS and em (2:06) I just felt this is something I have to give back

That lexical retrieval was not impaired in Samantha was further demonstrated by her semantic (category) fluency score of 21 animal names in 60 seconds. This score exceeds by 4 to 5 names **category fluency** scores obtained by subjects with MS in published studies.[25,26] In fact, Samantha's category fluency score is consistent with normative data for people of similar age, and exceeds mean scores obtained for people of the same educational background and gender.[27] Samantha's phonemic (letter) fluency score is 12 words in 60 seconds. This score is consistent with scores obtained for patients with MS in published studies.[25,26] It is also consistent with mean **letter fluency** scores for individuals without neurodegenerative disorder of the same gender as Samantha and slightly below mean scores for individuals of the same age and educational background as Samantha.[27] There is no evidence of impaired executive control based on Samantha's letter fluency performance. An association has been found between **pragmatics** (see below) and **verbal fluency** in MS.[28]

In terms of sentence **semantics**, Samantha was able to use a wide range of semantic or participant roles to characterise entities in a situation. These roles are associated with verbs and included patient, goal, experiencer, stimulus, **agent** and location, as in the following examples:

> a plant [PATIENT] seems to have fallen on his head [GOAL]
> you [EXPERIENCER] can imagine the colour [STIMULUS]
> the barn door [PATIENT] opened
> I [AGENT] was working in the kitchen [LOCATION]

Samantha's evident strengths in **morphology**, syntax and semantics were not consistently replicated by her performance in pragmatic and **discourse** aspects of language, however. Samantha did exhibit several intact pragmatic and discourse skills. This included the use of non-literal language as in the following examples of **hyperbole, idiom** and **metaphor**:

Hyperbole:

you wouldn't think of that <u>in a million years</u>

Idiom:

it didn't even <u>cross my mind</u> that much, relapses didn't happen that often sort of <u>fell down the ladder</u> in terms of priorities in people's minds

Metaphor:

the sky turned a bit em <u>angry</u> probably

There was limited opportunity to observe Samantha's understanding of **figurative language** during the session. The comprehension of some aspects of figurative language (e.g. metaphor) has been found to be impaired in MS.[29] However, Samantha did at least display intact comprehension of the idiom in the following utterance of the author:

INV: you can have a positive attitude but then you <u>hit the wall</u> of physical difficulties
SAM: you do hit the wall yeah

There was also some evidence that Samantha could undertake **conversational repair** as in the following example of self-initiated self-repair:

he had picked up that silver sorry that em glass slipper

These pragmatic aspects of language occurred alongside good turn-taking skills in conversation, the contribution of relevant and informative utterances to conversation, and appropriate use of **deixis**:

it was really good to see money <u>coming</u> in

(spatial deixis)

my fatigue levels weren't anything like what they are <u>now</u>

(temporal deixis)

In terms of **discourse**, Samantha drew at least one plausible **inference** when she remarked during her retelling of the Sam and Fred story that the weather was fine:

I think at the beginning of the story <u>the weather was fine</u>

She was also able to use a range of **cohesive devices** in conversation and other discourse contexts, as illustrated by these examples of **ellipsis, lexical substitution** and **anaphoric reference**:

Ellipsis:

INV: and did you enjoy that work?
SAM: I did [*enjoy that work*] it was wonderful

Lexical substitution:

I love seeing inside of homes and, and you know the price that they are and where they are and which <u>one</u> I would pick

Anaphoric reference:

INV: and do you miss <u>being in the workplace</u>?
SAM: I miss <u>it</u> because you miss the discipline of seeing everybody

Samantha's discourse abilities extended to the use of **direct reported speech**, a complex cognitive-linguistic skill that can promote listener engagement:[30]

> you know it's embarrassing because I remember the financial adviser, rang him and said "I've got this letter (.) em and I don't think it's good but I need your advice cause I don't know what I've to do here" and he says "well, can you read me the letter?" and I couldn't read the letter

However, alongside these areas of discourse strength were several discourse weaknesses. Even in the absence of marked cognitive decline and disability, people with MS have been found to have problems drawing inferences.[29,31,32] Samantha drew incorrect inferences during her narration of the Flowerpot Incident. This resulted in a misinterpretation of the events in the pictures. She inferred, for example, that the gentleman in the pictures entered his own home and that the woman who answered the door is the gentleman's wife. However, neither inference is plausible given other information that is provided in the pictures. If the man were entering his own home, he would not have to knock on the door with his walking stick to gain entry. Also, it is unlikely that the man would doff his hat to the woman and kiss her hand, both formal behaviours that suggest a lack of prior acquaintance, if the woman in the pictures were the gentleman's wife:

Flowerpot Incident:

> so, Tom is out with his little dog he's got a walking stick (.) am (.) and a plant seems to have fallen on his head (.) em (.) whether it's outside his home em (4:99) his dog seems to be quite alarmed at this and, and sort of has sort of stepped back (.) em but Tom's going to go into the house <u>must be his home</u> and with the dog um following and he slams the door behind him (.) <u>his wife's there</u> and she welcomes this little puppy or his little dog in to em (2:10) and the dog's got a bone and he runs away with it which <u>the wife has given him</u> and we're not quite sure what <u>the wife and husband are going to do now</u>

Consistent with her self-reported memory difficulties, Samantha could recall the details of the Sam and Fred story when these were part of a well-established script. In fact, she even refers to such a script when she states at the outset of her retelling that "it sounds like an Irish not that far away story". However, details in the story that could not be inferred from the script were evidently lacking in her narrative. This included the fact that Sam and Fred had farmed the land *for 30 years* and that the distressed farmers received assistance from *people in the local village*:

Sam and Fred (immediate recall):

> it sounds like an Irish not that far away story but it's about two brothers em Sam and Fred em we don't know their ages but they farmed the land together am both crop and animals they em (.) I think at the beginning of the story the weather was fine em but they had indications whether it was forecast or just being farmers knowing that there was going to be a turn in the weather em which happened a lot quicker than they were expecting the sky turned a bit em angry probably and I think opened and em (.) rained down very heavily so lots of crops were destroyed the barn door opened and the animals sheep and cattle escaped and it took them some time to round them all up again and em I think get them recovered em and they probably lost quite a lot of their crops

Memory difficulties might also explain one of two noteworthy features of Samantha's Cinderella narrative. Samantha was clearly unsure from memory, even after viewing the picture book, about the circumstances that had led to Cinderella living with her stepmother and stepsisters. This uncertainty was reflected in her extensive use of the hedge *sort of* in the early part of the story. In the first 119 words (or 36%) of her Cinderella narrative, Samantha used one instance of *sort of* every 23 words (e.g. "she sort of grew up there"). In the remaining two-thirds of the story that addressed more familiar events – Cinderella meets her fairy god-mother and attends the ball at the palace – there was not a single further instance of the hedge *sort of*. Samantha's uncertainty in her recall of the story is reflected in her use of **hedging**.

When Samantha was on more familiar ground in describing events at the ball, she was able to produce a very detailed narrative. However, her detailed narrative was abruptly terminated in a manner that violates listener expectations around narrative closure. The narrator must not only state that the glass slipper fitted Cinderella (as indeed Samantha does), but also indicate the significance of this fact. Its significance is that the prince had succeeded in identifying the mystery woman whom he had danced with at the ball and whom he intended to marry. The omission of this information means that there has been no explicit resolution to the earlier problem or dilemma in the story – the prince wanted to marry the woman he danced with but could not identify her. Samantha's premature termination of the story might suggest some additional discourse difficulty on her part with **story grammar**. The conclusion of Samantha's Cinderella narrative is shown below:

Cinderella narrative:

> so he went around all the houses in the countryside and in and around where the castle was that (.) people had come to the ball for and (.) he (.) had huge, huge task finding the owner of the slipper but he found eventually that it was Cinderella who owned it and they married happy ever after

COMMUNICATION PROFILE:

Speech intelligibility:

- Samantha displayed fully intelligible speech production; there was no motor speech disorder, either dysarthria or apraxia of speech; there was no evidence of phonological impairment.

Morphology and syntax:

- Samantha had intact morphology and used a wide range of inflectional and derivational morphemes; she was able to produce and understand complex syntax.

Vocabulary and semantics:

- Samantha displayed strong lexical-semantic skills; achieved 89% accuracy on confrontation naming, with her small number of errors semantically related to target words; no evidence of word-finding difficulty in conversation; semantic fluency score exceeded norms for MS clinical samples and was consistent with scores for people without neurodegenerative disorder; she used a range of semantic roles to characterise entities in sentences.

Pragmatics:

- Samantha was able to use non-literal language including hyperbole, metaphor and idiom; she understood indirect speech acts and was able to undertake conversational repair; took turns and used deixis appropriately; Samantha was able to contribute relevant, informative utterances to conversation and other types of discourse.

Discourse:

- Samantha had identifiable discourse deficits; she could draw plausible inferences but often drew inferences in discourse that resulted in misinterpretation of events; omitted information from narratives when it was not part of a well-established script; used hedging to express uncertainty during narrative production; there was some evidence of impaired knowledge of story grammar; she was able to use direct reported speech, mental state language and devices like ellipsis, anaphoric reference and lexical substitution to achieve cohesion in discourse.

Cognition:

- Samantha's category and letter fluency performances did not suggest lexical retrieval difficulties or problems with executive control; self-reported problems with memory were evident in the omission of information in narratives when she could not draw on a well-established script; Samantha appeared to need more time to plan the grammatical structure of utterances, as indicated by extensive use of fillers like *em* at syntactic boundaries.

Suggestions for Further Reading

(1) Murdoch, B. and Theodoros, D. (eds) (2000) *Speech and Language Disorders in Multiple Sclerosis.* London and Philadelphia: Whurr Publishers.

This edited volume is the only book dedicated to an examination of speech and language disorders in MS. The first section examines motor speech disorders in MS. This includes perceptual and acoustic features of dysarthria in MS, as well as impairments of speech production sub-systems such as articulation and phonation. The second section examines language disorder in MS in areas such as naming and discourse. The treatment of language disorders is also addressed.

(2) Carotenuto, A., Iodice, R. and Arcara, G. (2021) 'Multiple sclerosis', in L. Cummings (Ed.), *Handbook of Pragmatic Language Disorders: Complex and Underserved Populations.* Cham, Switzerland: Springer International Publishing AG, to appear.

This chapter examines pragmatic language impairments in people with MS and reports results from the authors' own investigations of this aspect of language. There is discussion of the neuroanatomical basis of pragmatic disorders in MS, the theory of mind and social cognitive impairments in this condition, and a review of the epidemiology, aetiology and pathophysiology of MS.

(3) Nota, A., Ganty, G., Lafortune, M., Vandevijver, A. and Vanlievendael, S. (2002) The Role of the Speech-Language Pathologist in the Rehabilitation of People with Multiple Sclerosis, Melsbroek, Belgium: National MS Centre. Accessed online on 9 February 2019: https://cdn.ymaws.com/www.mscare.org/resource/resmgr/Articles/Article0007_RoleofSLPinMS.pdf.

This document is produced by the Speech and Language Department of the National MS Centre in Belgium. It examines in some detail the assessment and management of dysarthria, swallowing and language disorders in MS, based on a review of the available evidence.

Questions

(1) During the sentence generation task, Samantha was given the words *child* and *hospital* and was asked to put them into a sentence. Her response is shown below. Based on your knowledge of her linguistic and cognitive difficulties, how would you characterise her response to this task?

> ah (2:64) em (5:32) ah, ah, ah (.) ah, ah, ah um (3:77) I do not like to see a child at the hospital

(2) One of Samantha's linguistic strengths was her ability to use a range of cohesive devices in conversation and other forms of discourse. What types of cohesion do the following extracts from her language sample exemplify?

   (a) **INV:** so that earlier work drew directly on your degree SAM: yes, it did
   (b) **SAM:** there's always three homes one's a mystery one
   (c) **SAM:** I literally can't bring my wee boy to school em I haven't had to on a few occasions my husband's had to do that as well
   (d) **SAM:** I'd made it out it took me probably an hour to do that when he said can I read it
   (e) **INV:** somehow you do manage SAM: you do it's amazing what you manage to do

(3) Samantha used mental state language throughout her language sample. Some extracts from this sample are shown below. For each extract: (i) identify the mental state(s) used; (ii) indicate if the mental state(s) is (are) cognitive or affective in nature; and (iii) indicate if the mental state(s) is (are) attributed to the speaker's mind or to the mind of another actor:

   (a) "I remember the neurologist saying to me "I don't think you'll be fit to deal with the heat" and I said "but it's not really an issue I've signed up to it I am going"
   (b) "the mother is preoccupied drying the dishes"
   (c) "I mean they've all been good we went to Florida"
   (d) "his dog seems to be quite alarmed"
   (e) "gosh I don't know this story at all"

(4) The adverb *there* can be used deictically (e.g. she collapsed *there*) and anaphorically (e.g. John bought a remote island and lived *there* for two years). Samantha made use of both deictic and anaphoric *there* in her language sample. Several utterances from her sample are listed below. For each utterance, indicate if she is making use of anaphoric *there*, deictic *there*, or both uses of the adverb:

   (a) "I don't know how I managed to go to work and spend all the hours and travel <u>there</u>"

(b) "I'm quite involved in our church where I would go down in and participate <u>there</u>"

(c) "I decided I was going to go on this em building a house building homes in Tanzania so I went over <u>there</u>"

(d) "her stepsisters headed off to the ball in their carriages and ah were famed to, to em find this prince that was going to be <u>there</u>"

(e) "I would have went in to promote self-employment […] and from <u>there</u> I em worked in a small company"

(f) "Tom's going to go into the house must be his home and with the dog um following and he slams the door behind him (.) his wife's <u>there</u>"

Answers

(1) Samantha's response to this task saw her produce a succession of fillers and three lengthy timed pauses. Samantha was clearly having difficulty planning and encoding an utterance that contained the target words *child* and *hospital*. The pauses and fillers provided Samantha with additional time to undertake the processing that is needed to encode her utterance which was well-formed when it was finally produced.

(2) (a) ellipsis: "yes, it did [*draw directly on my degree*]"

(b) lexical substitution: "there's always three homes <u>one</u>'s a mystery <u>one</u>"

(c) ellipsis: "I literally can't bring my wee boy to school em I haven't had to [*bring him to school*] on a few occasions my husband's had to do that as well"

(d) anaphoric reference: "<u>I'd made it out</u> it took me probably an hour to do <u>that</u> when he said can I read it"

(e) ellipsis: "you do [*manage*] it's amazing what you manage to do"

(3) (a) *remember* (cognitive): attributed to the speaker's mind; *think* (cognitive): attributed to the mind of another actor (neurologist)

(b) *preoccupied* (affective): attributed to the mind of another actor (mother)

(c) *mean* (cognitive): attributed to the speaker's mind

(d) *alarmed* (affective): attributed to the mind of another actor (dog)

(e) *know* (cognitive): attributed to the speaker's mind

(4) (a) *there* functions anaphorically in its reference to 'work', and deictically in that Samantha is indicating that she is not currently at work.

(b) *there* functions anaphorically in its reference to 'our church', and deictically in that Samantha is indicating that she is not currently at church.

(c) *there* functions anaphorically in its reference to 'Tanzania', and deictically in that Samantha is indicating that she is not currently in Tanzania.

(d) *there* functions anaphorically in its reference to 'the ball'.

(e) *there* functions anaphorically in its reference to 'promote self-employment'.

(f) *there* functions anaphorically in its reference to 'the house'.

References

[1] Wallin, M.T., Culpepper, W.J., Nichols, E., Bhutta, Z.A., Gebrehiwot, T.T., Hay, S.I., Khalil, I.A., Krohn, K.J., Liang, X., Naghavi, M., Mokdad, A.H., Nixon, M.R., Reiner, R.C., Sartorius, B., Smith, M., Topor-Madry, R., Werdecker, A., Vos, T., Feigin, V.L. and Murray, C.J.L. (2019) 'Global, regional, and national burden of multiple sclerosis 1990-2016: A systematic analysis for the Global Burden of Disease Study 2016', *Lancet Neurology*, 18 (3): 269–285.

[2] Wallin, M.T., Culpepper, W.J., Campbell, J.D., Nelson, L.M., Langer-Gould, A., Marrie, R.A., Cutter, G.R., Kaye, W.E., Wagner, L., Tremlett, H., Buka, S.L., Dilokthornsakul, P., Topol, B., Chen, L.H. and LaRocca, N.G. (2019) 'The prevalence of MS in the United States: A population-based estimate using health claims data', *Neurology*, 92 (10): e1029–e1040.

[3] Houzen, H., Niino, M., Hata, D., Nakano, F., Kikuchi, S., Fukazawa, T. and Sasaki, H. (2008). 'Increasing prevalence and incidence of multiple sclerosis in northern Japan', *Multiple Sclerosis Journal*, 14 (7), 887–892.

[4] Ascherio, A. and Munger, K.L. (2016) 'Epidemiology of multiple sclerosis: From risk factors to prevention-an update', *Seminars in Neurology*, 36 (2): 103–114.

[5] Lunde, H.M.B., Assmus, J., Myhr, K.M., Bø, L. and Grytten, N. (2017) 'Survival and cause of death in multiple sclerosis: A 60-year longitudinal population study', *Journal of Neurology, Neurosurgery, and Psychiatry*, 88 (8): 621–625.

[6] Stewart, T., Spelman, T., Havrdova, E. et al. for the MSBase Study Group (2017) 'Contribution of different relapse phenotypes to disability in multiple sclerosis', *Multiple Sclerosis*, 23 (2): 266–276.

[7] Merson, R.M. and Rolnick, M.I. (1998) 'Speech-language pathology and dysphagia in multiple sclerosis', *Physical Medicine and Rehabilitation Clinics of North America*, 9 (3): 631–641.

[8] Alali, D., Ballard, K. and Bogaardt, H. (2018) 'The frequency of dysphagia and its impact on adults with multiple sclerosis based on patient-reported questionnaires', *Multiple Sclerosis and Related Disorders*, 25: 227–231.

[9] Rao, S.M. (1995) 'Neuropsychology of multiple sclerosis', *Current Opinion in Neurology*, 8 (3): 216–220.

[10] DeSousa, E.A., Albert, R.H. and Kalman, B. (2002) 'Cognitive impairments in multiple sclerosis: A review', *American Journal of Alzheimer's Disease and Other Dementias*, 17 (1): 23–29.

[11] Patti, F. and Vila, C. (2014) 'Symptoms, prevalence and impact of multiple sclerosis in younger patients: A multinational survey', *Neuroepidemiology*, 42 (4): 211–218.

[12] Nazareth, T.A., Rava, A.R., Polyakov, J.L., Banfe, E.N., Waltrip II, R.W., Zerkowski, K.B. and Herbert, L.B. (2018) 'Relapse prevalence, symptoms, and health care engagement: Patient insights from the Multiple Sclerosis in America 2017 survey', *Multiple Sclerosis and Related Disorders*, 26: 219–234.

[13] Klugman, T.M. and Ross, E. (2002) 'Perceptions of the impact of speech, language, swallowing, and hearing difficulties on quality of life of a group of South African persons with multiple sclerosis', *Foila Phoniatrica et Logopaedica*, 54 (4): 201–221.

[14] Minden, S.L., Moes, E.J., Orav, J., Kaplan, E. and Reich, P. (1990) 'Memory impairment in multiple sclerosis', *Journal of Clinical and Experimental Neuropsychology*, 12 (4): 566–586.

[15] Thornton, A.E. and Raz, N. (1997) 'Memory impairment in multiple sclerosis: A quantitative review', *Neuropsychology*, 11 (3): 357–366.

[16] Siegert, R. and Abernethy, D. (2005) 'Depression in multiple sclerosis: A review', *Journal of Neurology, Neurosurgery & Psychiatry*, 76 (4): 469–475.

[17] Yorkston, K.M., Baylor, C. and Amtmann, D. (2014) 'Communicative participation restrictions in multiple sclerosis: Associated variables and correlation with social functioning', *Journal of Communication Disorders*, 52: 196–206.

[18] Noffs, G., Perera, T., Kolbe, S.C., Shanahan, C.J., Boonstra, F.M.C., Evans, A., Butzkueven, H., van der Walt, A. and Vogel, A.P. (2018) 'What speech can tell us: A systematic review of dysarthria characteristics in multiple sclerosis', *Autoimmunity Reviews*, 17: 1202–1209.

[19] Roberg, B.L., Somogie, M., Thelen, J.M. and Bruce, J.M. (2015) 'Articulation time does not affect speeded cognitive performance in multiple sclerosis', *Cognitive and Behavioral Neurology*, 28 (1): 33–38.

[20] Svindt, V., Bóna, J. and Hoffmann, I. (2020) 'Changes in temporal features of speech in secondary progressive multiple sclerosis (SPMS) – case studies', *Clinical Linguistics & Phonetics*, 34 (4): 339–356.

[21] Grossman, M., Robinson, K.M., Onishi, K., Thompson, H., Cohen, J. and D'Esposito, M. (1995) 'Sentence comprehension in multiple sclerosis', *Acta Neurologica Scandinavica*, 92 (4): 324–331.

[22] Kujala, P., Portin, R. and Ruutiainen, J. (1996) 'Language functions in incipient cognitive decline in multiple sclerosis', *Journal of the Neurological Sciences*, 141: 79–86.

[23] Friend, K.B., Rabin, B.M., Groninger, L., Deluty, R.H., Bever, C. and Grattan, L. (1999) 'Language functions in patients with multiple sclerosis', *The Clinical Neuropsychologist*, 13 (1): 78–94.

[24] Beatty, W.W. and Monson, N. (1989) 'Lexical processing in Parkinson's disease and multiple sclerosis', *Journal of Geriatric Psychiatry and Neurology*, 2 (3): 145–152.

[25] Jakimovski, D., Weinstock-Guttman, B., Roy, S., Jaworski III, M., Hancock, L., Nizinski, A., Srinivasan, P., Fuchs, T.A., Szigeti, K., Zivadinov, R. and Benedict, R.H.B. (2019) 'Cognitive profiles of aging in multiple sclerosis', *Frontiers in Aging Neuroscience*, 11: 105. doi: 10.3389/fnagi.2019.00105

[26] Beatty, W.W. (2002) 'Fluency in multiple sclerosis: Which measure is best?', *Multiple Sclerosis*, 8: 261–264.

[27] Tombaugh, T.N., Kozak, J. and Rees, L. (1999) 'Normative data stratified by age and education for two measures of verbal fluency: FAS and animal naming', *Archives of Clinical Neuropsychology*, 14 (2): 167–177.

[28] Carotenuto, A., Arcara, G., Orefice, G., Cerillo, I., Giannino, V., Rasulo, M., Iodice, R. and Bambini, V. (2018) 'Communication in multiple sclerosis: Pragmatic deficit and its relation with cognition and social cognition', *Archives of Clinical Neuropsychology*, 33 (2): 194–205.

[29] Lethlean, J.B. and Murdoch, B.E. (1997) 'Performance of subjects with multiple sclerosis on tests of high-level language', *Aphasiology*, 11 (1): 39–57.

[30] Cummings, L. (2016) 'Reported speech: A clinical pragmatic perspective', in A. Capone, F. Kiefer and F. Lo Piparo (eds), *Indirect Reports and Pragmatics*, Series: Perspectives in Pragmatics, Philosophy & Psychology, Vol. 5, Cham, Switzerland: Springer International Publishing AG, 31–55.

[31] Chanial, C., Basaglia-Pappas, S., Jacqueline, S., Boulange, A., Gourdon, C., Donya, S., Fagnou, S., Laurent, B., Camdessanche, J.-P. and Borg, C. (2020) 'Assessment of implicit language and theory of mind in multiple sclerosis', *Annals of Physical and Rehabilitation Medicine*, 63: 111–115.

[32] Barwood, C.H.S. and Murdoch, B.E. (2013) 'Cognitive linguistic deficits in relapsing-remitting multiple sclerosis', *Aphasiology*, 27 (12): 1459–1471.

CASE STUDY 6

Parkinson's Disease

KEY FACTS AND FIGURES:

- Parkinson's disease (PD) is the second most common neurodegenerative disorder after Alzheimer's disease. It is caused by the depletion of cells in the substantia nigra of the brain that produce the neurotransmitter substance dopamine. The cell loss occurs in association with the formation of Lewy bodies.
- In 2016, 6.1 million people globally had PD, an increase from 2.5 million in 1990.[1] There were 680,000 individuals aged ≥45 years with PD in the United States in 2010, a prevalence of 572 per 100,000.[2] Prevalence increases with age from 41 per 100,000 in 40 to 49 years to 1,087 per 100,000 in 70 to 79 years.[3] Annual incidence rates in ten European countries range from 5 per 100,000 to 346 per 100,000.[4] A male-to-female ratio of 1.6:1 is reported.[5]
- Genetic, environmental and behavioural factors are known to modify the risk of PD. An increased risk of PD is associated with exposure to pesticides, consumption of dairy products, history of melanoma and traumatic brain injury. A reduced risk of PD is associated with smoking, caffeine consumption, higher serum urate concentrations, physical activity, and use of ibuprofen and other medications.[6]
- Life expectancy in PD and age at time of death vary with age of onset. Mean life expectancy is 38 years for onset between 25 and 39 years, 21 years for onset between 40 and 64 years, and 5 years for onset ≥65 years. Average age at time of death is 71 years for onset between 25 and 39

DOI: 10.4324/9781003153559-7

years (82 years in general population), and 88 years for individuals ≥65
years (91 years in general population).[7]
- The cardinal motor symptoms in PD are tremor, bradykinesia (slowness
  of movement) and rigidity. Non-motor symptoms include cognitive
  impairments, neuropsychiatric symptoms like depression and anxiety,
  autonomic disorders such as gastrointestinal and urinary symptoms,
  sleep disturbances and pain.

Background

Frank (not his real name) is 61;8 years old. He was diagnosed with PD in May
2006. Frank is married and has three grown-up children, two sons and a daughter. All three of his children live locally to him. He has five grandchildren, three
grandsons and two granddaughters. Frank is a former building contractor who
worked on house construction. He left school at 16 years of age and worked
for his brother for 32 years. He retired at the age of 48 years. Frank first became
aware that all was not well in 1992. There was a lack of movement in his left
arm. It was also stiff and would not swing freely. Over time, his left leg was also
affected. He developed a lack of facial expression. Frank visited his GP complain-
ing of pain in his left arm but both he and his doctor attributed this to an injury
he had sustained at work. For five years between 1997 and 2002, Frank made
many visits to his doctor, but no answers were forthcoming about the symptoms
he was experiencing. In 2004, Frank visited a different doctor privately who
thought his problems were caused by hardening of the arteries in his neck. He
was advised to consult a neurologist. In January 2005, Frank was referred by his
doctor to a consultant at a sports injuries clinic at a regional hospital. He was
seen by the consultant in February 2005 and was referred to physiotherapy. The
physiotherapist assessed Frank in March 2005 but could not find any problems
to work on.

Between November 2005 and February 2006, Frank attended a Chinese
clinic where he received 18 weekly sessions of acupuncture in his arm and back
with a view to alleviating the pain he was experiencing. In February 2006, Frank
had an operation on his knee. He was 40 years old at the time. The pain and
movement problems in his left arm were getting worse. The left side of his body
was out of alignment and he had difficulty holding a fork when eating. His vision
was affected when he turned his head to reverse a vehicle. When his eyes were
shut, he had difficulty making finger-to-nose movements. In March 2006, Frank
visited a consultant neurologist privately. An MRI scan and urine test for Wilson's
disease were conducted. In May 2006, Frank had another MRI scan and PD
was diagnosed. Frank was under the care of a private neurologist between May
2006 and 2010. He was on medication during this time. However, his condition

was progressively deteriorating. He had falls, involuntary movements, some falls related to blackouts, freezing episodes and constipation.

In 2011, Frank was referred to the National Health Service and was placed under the care of three consultant neurologists. During a 2-week hospital stay, an **apomorphine** pump was fitted. In 2012, Frank developed dyskinesia following a 2-week stay in hospital. The apomorphine pump controlled these involuntary movements. However, by the end of June 2016 the pump was no longer controlling Frank's symptoms and he was unable to sit, stand or walk. In July 2016 Frank was admitted to hospital to have the apomorphine pump removed. A **Duopa** pump was fitted in September 2016 and the medical staff and physiotherapists tried to get Frank on his feet again. By December 2016, Frank had still not been able to get back onto his feet. Frank's wife reported that his extended bed rest in hospital had a very negative effect on him. In January 2017, Frank was transferred to the neurology ward in a different hospital. There they tried to get Frank onto his feet, but it was not very successful. When Frank returned home in March 2017, he was able to move and help his wife and carers a little. By 2018, Frank was making permanent use of his wheelchair. His wife reported that his mood could get very low. With increased immobility, constipation became a growing problem for Frank. Between August and December 2019, Frank had three periods of hospitalisation to treat a blockage in his bowel. Frank's bowel problems have left him feeling unwell. He tends to sleep a lot and is unresponsive to those around him.

Frank is currently seeing his neurologist approximately every 4 months. He has no family history of PD. In December 2001, he was physically assaulted and was badly kicked around the head. Two of Frank's teeth were knocked out during the attack, and he required 11 stitches. Head trauma is a risk factor for PD.[8] Prior to his PD diagnosis, Frank enjoyed several active pursuits. He was an avid skier, undertaking 19 skiing trips to countries such as France, Andorra, Italy, Austria and Bulgaria. Each trip lasted a week and he took skiing lessons. Frank also owned a boat for 12 years, although he had not been on it for nearly 3 years by the time of the author's visit. He participated in rally car racing, only retiring in 2011 when he began to have difficulty getting out of the car. He was the navigator in the car and participated in competitions all round Ireland such as the national rally championships. Frank enjoys watching television. His favourite channels are Discovery and Quest. He particularly enjoys programmes to do with big machines. He explained that this is because he worked as a mechanical fitter for four years and made parts for turbines. He left this job to work for his brother.

Clinical Symptoms

Frank displays very little movement. He is unable to walk and has poor balance. He uses a wheelchair permanently. Frank's concentration is poor at times. His ability to plan is also compromised and his **attention** can deteriorate after a short time. His wife reports his **memory** to be good. Frank's sleep, appetite, continence and swallowing have all been affected by PD. Constipation is a significant and ongoing problem for Frank. He was hospitalised for two nights in August 2019 to treat a blockage in his bowel. The procedure was repeated in September 2019 and again in December 2019. Frank also experiences **depression**. His wife reports a reduction in his sense of smell, a recognised symptom of PD.[9]

Daily Activities

Frank's wife reports that every aspect of his life has been adversely affected by PD. This includes family duties and responsibilities, leisure activities, hobbies and interests, social activities and friendship networks, driving, work and the ability to undertake household tasks. The impact on family life has been particularly profound. Frank's wife states that:

> our children and grandchildren have really lost out on a great father and grandfather who would have been a great source of help to all of them in their lives and as you know with [Frank] being a builder he could have been helping the family with so much. I think this is really the hardest thing for him.

Frank is dependent on his wife and carers for all aspects of his personal care. Two carers visit him four times every day and assist him with toileting, dressing and bathing.

Medication

In 2011, Frank had a 2-week hospital stay during which time an apomorphine pump was fitted. By the end of June 2016, the pump was no longer working as Frank could not sit, stand or walk. In September 2016, a Duopa pump was fitted during a 1-month hospital stay. Frank takes other medications to treat his PD symptoms. This includes Madopar CR capsules, gabapentin 300 mg capsules and baclofen 10 mg tablets. Frank has been prescribed senna 7.5 mg tablets and Laxido Orange oral powder to treat constipation, mirtazapine 30 mg tablets to treat depression, and clonazepam 500 microgram tablets to treat sleep problems. Frank has several other medical problems that require medication. He takes atorvastatin 20 mg tablets to treat high cholesterol, amlodipine 5 mg tablets for high blood pressure, aspirin 75 mg tablets to thin his blood, and Janumet 50/1,000 mg tablets to treat diabetes. Frank has been prescribed a range of vitamin and mineral tablets, including Vitamin B compound strong tablets, thiamine (vitamin B1) 100 mg tablets, ascorbic acid (vitamin C) 50 mg tablets, fultium-D3 800 unit (vitamin D) capsules, and ferrous sulphate (iron) 200 mg tablets.

Communication

Frank's wife reports that PD has affected the **intelligibility** of his speech. She states that he speaks with a slower speech rate and reduced speech volume. The **fluency** of his speech is also compromised. Frank's **voice quality** is described as "breathy" by his wife. Frank's first appointment with speech and language therapy is scheduled for March 2020. He has been on the waiting list for therapy for over two years.

The author visited Frank at home on the morning of 3 August 2018. His wife was present throughout the visit. We worked at a large table in the dining area adjacent to the kitchen. Frank sat in his wheelchair at the head of the table and his wife and the author sat to either side of him. For tasks that required Frank to look at pictures, his wife put his glasses on for him. For other activities, the glasses were removed. A display stand was used for all visual materials so that Frank was not attempting to look at pictures that were flat on the table. Two short breaks were taken during the session. One break was prompted by the arrival of Frank's carers to take him to the toilet. Frank was responsive, attentive and cooperative throughout the recording. He did not fatigue and undertook all tasks as requested. The visit concluded just at the point when Frank's daughter and grandchildren pulled into the driveway in their car.

Frank exhibited intelligible speech production during the session. However, there appeared to be speech motoric influences on sentence complexity. (The exact relationship between **motor speech production** and language in PD is an issue of some contention.[10]) Frank had limited breath support for speech. He spoke in short, truncated utterances as his breathing would permit. He often omitted words to conserve his breath such as the **personal pronoun** 'I' in utterances like "used to do grant work" and "always took lessons". He could also occasionally be heard running out of breath towards the end of utterances. Because he spoke in short utterances, his speech lacked normal **intonation** and was monotone, as is typical of **hypokinetic dysarthria** in PD.[11,12] Frank's **resonance** was in the normal range and his **voice quality** was slightly breathy. His rate of speech was increased as he tried to say as much as possible before running out of breath. This finding of increased speech rate is consistent with previous studies.[13,14] Frank's speech contained numerous pauses which affected his **fluency**. Pauses were needed to replenish the expiratory airflow for speech and to plan his utterances. There was no evidence of **apraxia of speech** or phonological impairment in Frank's speech. During the test session, Frank did not use **gestures** or facial expressions, both of which are known to be impaired in PD.[15,16]

Frank's expressive language was well formed for the most part. He used a wide range of inflectional and derivational morphemes, as these examples illustrate:

Inflectional morphemes:

> entail<u>ed</u>; turbine<u>s</u>; bigg<u>est</u> thing; doctor<u>'s</u> office; go<u>ing</u>

Derivational morphemes:

> <u>re</u>aligning; build<u>ing</u> contract<u>or</u>; mechanic<u>al</u> fitt<u>er</u>

Although his utterances were short, Frank was able to express a range of **clauses**, including infinitive, relative and *-ing* participle clauses:

> I had [to take my child to the hospital]
>
> > (*infinitive*)

> I have a tree [growing in my garden]
>
> > (*-ing participle clause*)

> two brothers (.) [who farmed the same (.) piece of land]
>
> > (*relative clause*)

Negative, interrogative and **passive voice** constructions were also used by Frank, albeit sparingly on account of his use of short utterances:

> I could<u>n't</u> get out of the car
>
> > (*negative*)

> <u>Wh</u>at do you call (.) Discovery?
>
> > (*interrogative*)

> I <u>was stuck</u> in it
>
> > (*passive voice*)

Frank was also able to comprehend utterances with complex **syntax** in conversation, including these examples of a **relative clause** (REL) in a yes-no interrogative and an interrogative **subordinate clause** (INT) in an imperative:

> Do you have any interests and hobbies [$_{REL}$that you enjoy pursuing in your free time]?
> Tell Louise [$_{INT}$what you served your time as]

Frank appeared to need additional time in which to plan the grammatical structure of his utterances. This is suggested by the lengthy pause(s) that preceded each utterance he produced during the sentence-generation task. **Executive function** deficits are a feature of PD, even in its early stage.[17] That these deficits may be compromising Frank's **planning** of utterances is suggested by his poor **phonemic fluency** score (see below). Although Frank displayed slowed **planning**, he was able to produce a well-formed utterance for each set of target words, as the following example illustrates:

INV: the three words are chair, doctor and sit
FRA: (13:83)
INV: chair, doctor and sit
FRA: (5:21) when I go to his clinic (.) I sit in the doctor's chair

Syntactic production and comprehension deficits do not appear to be inevitable in PD. Individuals with PD and no **dementia** have been found not to have syntactic production deficits despite having impairments in **lexical retrieval**, repetition of words and sentences, and speech production.[18] PD patients with no dementia have low comprehension error rates that are similar to those of healthy individuals, with high comprehension error rates only evident in mildly demented PD patients.[19] Although Frank has some mild cognitive difficulties, as indicated by his poor phonemic fluency performance, these difficulties appear not to have a detrimental effect on his expressive and receptive **syntax**.

Lexical-semantic impairments are commonly reported in PD, with evidence of superior processing of concrete nouns over action verbs.[20–22] Frank's lexical-semantic skills were an area of relative strength. He named all but two items correctly in the **confrontation naming** task (a third item, *ostrich*, was named as 'emu' and was judged to be correct). Frank was inconsistent in his response to phonemic and **semantic cues**. Both types of cue successfully elicited production of 'French horn'. However, neither cue was effective in eliciting production of 'pumpkin':

Target 'French horn':

FRA: (6:18) dunno what it is
INV: okay it's a type of musical instrument
FRA: yes
INV: a fr, fr, French
FRA: French horn

Target 'pumpkin':

INV: this is something that people carve during the Halloween holidays
FRA: yes

INV: begins with a pah
FRA: (2:93)
INV: you can make soup out of it, I've never made soup out of it, but it does make tasty soup, it's a pah, pump
FRA: (3:97)
INV: pump, kin
FRA: pumpkin

There was no evidence that Frank experienced **word-finding difficulty** in conversation. That Frank's lexical retrieval skills were reasonably intact was also suggested by his **semantic fluency** score. Frank produced 16 animal names in 60 seconds. This score is only slightly below the mean semantic fluency scores of healthy individuals who are the same age (17.6 names) and gender (17.4 names) and have the same educational background (16.7 names) as Frank.[23] Frank's semantic fluency score is consistent with mean scores obtained in clinical samples of individuals with PD.[24,25] Frank obtained a phonemic (letter) fluency score of 5 words beginning with the letter F in 60 seconds. This is significantly lower than mean **letter fluency** scores obtained by healthy individuals of similar age (12.8 words), gender (12.3 words) and educational background (12.2 words) to Frank.[23] It is also lower than mean letter fluency scores in clinical samples of individuals with PD.[25,26] Frank's poor phonemic fluency performance, and much stronger semantic fluency performance, suggests **executive dysfunction** in the absence of lexical retrieval impairment.

Because Frank spoke in short, truncated utterances, there were few instances of his use of conjunctions to link **clauses** according to complex meaning relations. Where normally the Cinderella narrative is an occasion for narrators to express relations like causation and consequence between events, Frank used the simple additive conjunction 'and' three times in the very short narrative that he produced (see below). Frank used several participant or **semantic roles** in the utterances he produced, including **agent**, patient, goal, source and location:

> a flowerpot [PATIENT] fell on his head [GOAL]
> it [PATIENT] came off a first-floor balcony [SOURCE]
> a man [AGENT] was walking up the street [LOCATION]

Frank displayed several intact pragmatic and **discourse** skills. He was able to take turns in conversation with the author and his wife. He contributed relevant, informative utterances to conversation and used laughter appropriately. **Speech act** comprehension has been found to be impaired in PD.[27] However, Frank used a range of speech acts in his own expressive language (e.g. seeking confirmation) and successfully identified the speech acts of others. For example, during his telling of the Flowerpot Incident, Frank was able to identify that the gentleman entered the building to *remonstrate* with the owner of the apartment from which the flowerpot fell, and that the elderly woman wanted to *make amends* for the injury that her flowerpot had caused:

> he decided to go upstairs (.) to give off
>
> > (speech act: *to remonstrate*)
>
> she'd (.) a bone for his dog (6:50) and that made things better
>
> > (speech act: *to make amends*)

Frank was able to participate in **conversational repair**. In these examples, he undertakes self-initiated self-repair with a view to providing his hearer with more specific information:

> put your name and address top corner, top right corner
> served my time as a fitter, mechanical fitter

Frank was also able to identify when he needed to correct a misunderstanding on the part of his hearer. His corrections were more skilled than simply repeating what he had said. Frank could have corrected the author (INV) by saying "no, skiing holidays" for his second turn in the exchange below. Instead, he opts for a less direct form of correction in his third turn by saying he had been away 19 times, from which the author could infer that he had undertaken more than one skiing holiday:

INV: can you maybe describe for me a holiday that you've had in the past that you've really enjoyed?
FRA: skiing holidays
INV: oh, a skiing holiday
FRA: yes
INV: wow when was this?
FRA: I was away 19 times
INV: 19 times

Frank's correction of his own utterances to address the informational needs of his hearer, and his correction of the utterances of others, suggests that he is adept at monitoring the belief states of his interlocutors in conversation. This mindreading ability gives some grounds for confidence that Frank has intact **theory of mind** (ToM) skills. ToM is a cognitive ability that can be impaired in PD even in the absence of **dementia**, leading to impairments in the comprehension of irony and other aspects of **pragmatics**.[28,29]

PD speakers have been reported to use incomplete and erroneous cohesive ties in narratives.[30] However, Frank displayed skilled use of **cohesion** across all discourse types. **Cohesive devices** such as **reference** (cataphoric and anaphoric), **ellipsis** and lexical reiteration were used appropriately to relate utterances to each other in conversation and other forms of discourse:

Cataphoric reference:

>   when I go to <u>his</u> clinic (.) I sit in the <u>doctor's</u> chair

Anaphoric reference:

>   served <u>my time as a fitter</u>, mechanical fitter making parts for turbines, so I did (.) spent four years at that first and left <u>there</u> soon as I finished (.) my time went to work for my brother then

>   case (.) something happened <u>the car</u> I was stuck in <u>it</u>

Ellipsis:

>   **INV:** are you happy enough to turn them [the pages] yourself?
>   **FRA:** I am [*happy enough to turn them myself*]

Lexical reiteration:

>   I've (.) set myself a <u>challenge</u> to (.) walk into the doctor's office in (.) Belfast City (.) he said I would never walk again (.) I'm going to prove him wrong (.) so that's what my <u>goal</u> is

Notwithstanding these pragmatic and discourse strengths, Frank did experience marked difficulty in the management of information in discourse. It was described above how Frank repaired his utterances when he judged that they were not sufficiently informative for his hearer. He also produced utterances like the following in which he volunteered more specific information unprompted by his interlocutor:

>   I was a building contractor, actually, house building

On other occasions, however, the author had to encourage Frank to produce the specific information that was required. This is evident in the following extract of conversation. The author asks Frank if he has a favourite TV programme, only to be given the name of a TV channel. The author must then ask a follow-up question to get the specific information she requires:

INV: do you have a favourite TV programme?
FRA: Discovery
INV: oh, the Discovery channel
FRA: yes
INV: right, so what sort of programmes on the Discovery channel do you like?

Occasionally, Frank presented incorrect information in discourse. During the Flowerpot Incident, he reported incorrectly that the gentleman "shook hands with the lady" when in fact he kissed the woman's hand. Frank also introduced information late during this discourse production task. The dog was mentioned for the first time at the end of the story even though it was pictured at the outset of the story, walking along the street with the gentleman:

> this woman come out (5:03) and she'd (.) a bone for <u>his dog</u>

But by far the most significant problem Frank had with information management during **discourse** was the omission of information. This was most evident when he was reliant on **memory** to produce a narrative or other type of discourse. Frank's immediate recall of the 100-word Sam and Fred story was particularly compromised. His narrative after a first and second reading contained little more than the names of the farmers and that they had worked together for many years:

Immediate recall after first reading:

> can't remember the name of, one was Sam (.) can't remember the other man's name (2:35) wer, wer, wer (*unintelligible*) (9:37) I can't remember anything else

Immediate recall after second reading:

> Sam and Fred were two farm, two brothers (.) who farmed the same (.) piece of land (.) for many years (10:96) that's it

However, these initial readings were not in vain and enabled Frank to develop a representation of the events in the story. Even though this representation was not sufficiently well formed to assist his immediate recall of the story, it did facilitate his delayed recall of the story at the end of the test session. Frank's narrative on delayed recall mentioned the adverse weather (rain), the fact that the door of the barn (shed) was blown open and the animals escaped, and that people from the

local village came to the farmers' assistance. None of this information was conveyed during immediate recall:

Delayed recall:

INV: Sam and Fred can you tell me any of that story back again?
FRA: (2:89) they were standing in the shed when it started to rain (2:88) and the
door burst open (.) all the cattle (.) sheep got out was (.) people in the (.)
next village (.) came and helped them round them up (3:71) that's it

That memory problems contributed to Frank's omission of information is also
supported by his performance on the Cinderella narrative task. This task requires
recall of a well-known fairy tale that is most often encountered for the first time in
childhood. It is useful to compare performance on this task, which involves reac-
tivation of an 'old' script, with the Sam and Fred story that assesses recall of newly
presented information. Once again, Frank omitted all but the most central details
of the story, suggesting that different types of memory may be problematic for him:

Cinderella narrative:

dunno the start of it she went to the ball (.) she lost her slipper (5:15) and
ah (3:49) prince found it and he took it back to her (3:89) and lived happily ever after

When Frank received pictorial support during a discourse production task, and
was not reliant on memory, he was able to produce an informative narrative. The
detail in both his narration of the Flowerpot Incident and his description of the
Cookie Theft picture is in stark contrast to his omission of information when
discourse production proceeded from memory:

Flowerpot Incident:

a man was walking up the street (.) when suddenly a flowerpot fell on his
head (.) it came off a first-floor balcony, so he decided to go upstairs (.) to
give off (.) he knocked on the door rather wildly (.) and this woman come
out (5:03) and she'd (.) a bone for his dog (6:50) and that made things better (3:08) he'd a right bump on his head (2:08) but he shook hands with
the lady (2:28) everyone was okay after that

Cookie Theft picture description:

two, two children (*unintelligible*) cookie jar (.) standing on a stool (.) it's
about to fall over (2:18) the mother she's washing dishes (.) ah, ah, dish (.)
she's drying the dishes (.) the water's running into the sink and running
over, over the floor and a nice day outside (4:06) that's it

Working memory deficits are well documented in PD[31–33] and have been linked with impaired pragmatic interpretation (e.g. **metaphor**) and problems in discourse production and comprehension.[34,35] Frank's memory–related discourse problems are, therefore, consistent with earlier findings.

COMMUNICATION PROFILE:

Speech intelligibility:

- Frank's speech production was fully intelligible; his respiratory support for speech was less than optimal, resulting in the production of short utterances, with some loss of volume for the articulation of utterance-final speech sounds; speech was monotonous as a normal intonational contour was not possible in Frank's truncated utterances; there was no evidence of apraxia of speech or phonological impairment.

Morphology and syntax:

- Frank's expressive language was well formed; he used the full range of inflectional and derivational morphemes; Frank produced different types of clauses, negation, interrogatives and passive voice constructions; he was also able to comprehend utterances with complex syntax; Frank appeared to need additional time in which to plan the grammatical structure of his utterances.

Vocabulary and semantics:

- Confrontation naming was an area of strength for Frank; semantic and phonemic cues occasionally prompted production of target words; no evidence of word-finding difficulty in conversation; Frank's semantic fluency score was slightly below normative values for healthy individuals of the same age, gender and educational background and was consistent with scores obtained in PD clinical samples; Frank made limited use of conjunctions that expressed complex conceptual relations like causation and consequence; he used a range of semantic or participant roles.

Pragmatics:

- Frank used language effectively for the most part; he took turns in conversation, contributed relevant, informative utterances and used laughter appropriately; he was able to use deixis and a range of speech acts; Frank engaged in conversational repair of his own utterances and used indirect means of correcting misunderstandings in his interlocutor; Frank was able to monitor his listener's beliefs and state of knowledge and adjust his utterances accordingly; Frank did not use gestures or facial expressions.

Discourse:

- Frank used a range of cohesive devices appropriately in discourse; his management of information varied significantly across different types of discourse, with omission of information most evident when he produced discourse from memory; occasionally, Frank produced incorrect information or introduced information late into discourse; when he had pictorial support, Frank could produce detailed, informative narratives and other forms of discourse.

Cognition:

- Frank's phonemic fluency score was lower than normative values based on healthy individuals and lower than values obtained in PD clinical samples, suggesting a significant executive function deficit; Frank's immediate recall of verbal material was very poor, while delayed recall was stronger; memory difficulties compromised discourse production; Frank displayed theory of mind skills as evidenced by his ability to read the intent of characters in narratives and by the occasional use of mental state language (e.g. "I was *scared* of anything happening").

Suggestions for Further Reading

(1) Theodoros, D. and Ramig, L. (eds) (2011) *Communication and Swallowing in Parkinson Disease*. San Diego, CA: Plural Publishing.

   This edited volume is the only book-length treatment of communication and swallowing in Parkinson's disease. The seven chapters examine symptoms and medical management of PD, speech, cognitive-linguistic and swallowing disorders in PD, and the neuropathology, assessment and treatment of communication and swallowing disorders in PD.

(2) Murray, L.L. (2008) 'Language and Parkinson's disease', *Annual Review of Applied Linguistics*, 28: 113–127.

   This wide-ranging review of language abilities in PD gives much needed focus to this often neglected aspect of the disorder. The author examines quantitative and qualitative changes in morphosyntax, lexical-semantic and discourse levels of language in PD.

(3) Miller, N. (2017) 'Communication changes in Parkinson's disease', *Practical Neurology*, 17 (4): 266–274.

The author conducts an extensive review of the communication changes that occur in PD, including speech and voice disorder, dysprosody and cognitive-linguistic impairments. The impact of these changes on mood and social participation is discussed. Approaches to assessment and directions for intervention are also considered.

Questions

(1) What is the discourse function of the underlined word in the following utterance that Frank produced during his conversation with the author?

> served my time as a fitter, mechanical fitter making parts for turbines, so I did (.) spent four years at <u>that</u> first and left there soon as I finished (.) my time went to work for my brother then

(2) It was stated above that Frank uses a range of speech acts in his expressive language. For the extracts below, identify the *type* of speech act that Frank is performing with each of his utterances:

Extract A:

INV: when were you last out on the boat Frank?
FRA: few year ago now, wasn't it (.) two years
WIF: be over two, three years nearly

Extract B:

INV: so, after all those skiing trips you must have actually become a very skilled skier
FRA: not really

Extract C:

FRA: what do you call (.) Discovery
WIF: Quest
FRA: Quest

Extract D:

INV: can you describe the type of work that you did before you retired?
FRA: I was a building contractor

Extract E:

FRA: he [the doctor] said I would never walk again (.) I'm going to prove
him wrong

(3) There was a marked difference in the informativeness of the different types
of discourse that Frank produced. When he recalled a story, even a short
story, from memory, considerable information was omitted. However, when
Frank had pictorial support during discourse production, he produced an
informative narrative that contained considerable detail. The Flowerpot
Incident was one such narrative. Examine this narrative, which is reproduced
below for convenience. Then answer the questions that follow.

> a man was walking up the street (.) when suddenly a flowerpot fell on
> his head (.) it came off a first-floor balcony, so he decided to go upstairs
> (.) to give off (.) he knocked on the door rather wildly (.) and this
> woman come out (5:03) and she'd (.) a bone for his dog (6:50) and that
> made things better (3:08) he'd a right bump on his head (2:08) but he
> shook hands with the lady (2:28) everyone was okay after that

(a) One way in which a story teller can make a narrative more vivid is by
including adverbs of manner that convey the speed and force of actions.
Identify *two* such adverbs in Frank's narrative.
(b) Frank's narrative is cohesive on account of his use of personal and
demonstrative pronouns to achieve anaphoric reference. Give *one* example of each type of anaphoric reference.
(c) Frank is adept at reading the intentional states of the two protagonists in
the story. Identify *two* instances where this occurs.
(d) As well as using anaphoric reference, Frank uses lexical reiteration to
achieve cohesion. Identify where this occurs in his narrative.
(e) There are several lengthy pauses in Frank's narrative. Where do these
pauses occur? What *two* factors may account for these pauses?

Answers

(1) The demonstrative pronoun *that* is used anaphorically to refer to 'mechanical fitter'.
(2) Each speech act is indicated in italics:
Extract A: Frank is using his utterance to *seek confirmation* from his wife.
Extract B: Frank is using his utterance to *deny* or *reject* what the author has
said.

Extract C: Frank is using his first utterance to *ask a question* and his second utterance to *provide confirmation.*

Extract D: Frank is using his utterance to *make an assertion.*

Extract E: Frank is *vowing* to prove his doctor wrong.

(3) (a) adverbs: suddenly; rather wildly

(b) personal pronoun: "<u>a flowerpot</u> fell on his head (.) <u>it</u> came off a first-floor balcony" demonstrative pronoun: "she'd (.) <u>a bone</u> for his dog (6:50) and <u>that</u> made things better"

(c) Frank can discern that the man wants to remonstrate ("to give off") with the owner of the apartment, and that the woman wants to make amends ("made things better") to the man for the injury he has sustained.

(d) lexical reiteration: "this <u>woman</u> come out ... he shook hands with the <u>lady</u>"

(e) The timed pauses arise at syntactic boundaries between clauses, e.g. "this woman come out (5:03) and she'd (.) a bone for his dog (6:50) and that made things better". This use of pauses may be explained by Frank's limited breath support for speech and by his need for additional time in which to plan his utterances.

References

[1] Dorsey, E.R., Elbaz, A., Nichols, E. et al. for the GBD 2016 Parkinson's Disease Collaborators (2018) 'Global, regional, and national burden of Parkinson's disease, 1990–2016: A systematic analysis for the Global Burden of Disease Study 2016', *Lancet Neurology*, 17 (11): 939–953.

[2] Marras, C., Beck, J.C., Bower, J.H., Roberts, E., Ritz, B., Ross, G.W., Abbott, R.D., Savica, R., Van Den Eeden, S.K., Willis, A.W., Tanner, C.M. on behalf of the Parkinson's Foundation P4 Group (2018) 'Prevalence of Parkinson's disease across North America', *NPJ Parkinson's Disease*, 4, 21. doi:10.1038/s41531-018-0058-0

[3] Pringsheim, T., Jette, N., Frolkis, A. and Steeves, T.D. (2014) 'The prevalence of Parkinson's disease: A systematic review and meta-analysis', *Movement Disorders*, 29 (13): 1583–1590.

[4] Von Campenhausen, S., Bornschein, B., Wick, R., Bötzel, K., Sampaio, C., Poewe, W., Oertel, W., Siebert, U., Berger, K. and Dodel, R. (2005) 'Prevalence and incidence of Parkinson's disease in Europe', *European Neuropsychopharmacology*, 15 (4): 473–490.

[5] Lubomski, M., Rushworth, R.L., Lee, W., Bertram, K.L. and Williams, D.R. (2014) 'Sex differences in Parkinson's disease', *Journal of Clinical Neuroscience*, 21 (9): 1503–1506.

[6] Ascherio, A. and Schwarzschild, M.A. (2016) 'The epidemiology of Parkinson's disease: Risk factors and prevention', *The Lancet Neurology*, 15 (12): 1257–1272.

[7] Ishihara, L.S., Cheesbrough, A., Brayne, C. and Schrag, A. (2007) 'Estimated life expectancy of Parkinson's patients compared with the UK population', *Journal of Neurology, Neurosurgery & Psychiatry*, 78 (12): 1304–1309.

[8] Gardner, R.C., Byers, A.L., Barnes, D.E., Li, Y., Boscardin, J. and Yaffe, K. (2018) 'Mild TBI and risk of Parkinson disease: A chronic effects of neurotrauma consortium study', *Neurology*, 90 (20): e1771–e1779. doi:10.1212/WNL0000000000005522.

[9] Hughes, K.C., Gao, X., Baker, J.M., Stephen, C., Kim, I.Y., Valeri, L. Schwarzschild, M.A. and Ascherio, A. (2018) 'Non-motor features of Parkinson's disease in a nested case-control study of US men', *Journal of Neurology, Neurosurgery, and Psychiatry*, 89 (12): 1288–1295.

[10] Auclair-Ouellet, N., Lieberman, P. and Monchi, O. (2017) 'Contribution of language studies to the understanding of cognitive impairment and its progression over time in Parkinson's disease', *Neuroscience and Biobehavioral Reviews*, 80: 657–672.

[11] Penner, H., Miller, N., Hertrich, I., Ackermann, H. and Schumm, F. (2001) 'Dysprosody in Parkinson's disease: An investigation of intonation patterns', *Clinical Linguistics & Phonetics*, 15 (7): 551–566.

[12] Ma, J.K.-Y., Schneider, C.B., Hoffmann, R. and Storch, A. (2015) 'Speech prosody across stimulus types for individuals with Parkinson's disease', *Journal of Parkinson's Disease*, 5: 291–299.

[13] Solomon, N.P. and Hixon, T.J. (1993) 'Speech breathing in Parkinson's disease', *Journal of Speech, Language, and Hearing Research*, 36 (2): 294–310.

[14] Skodda, S. (2011) 'Aspects of speech rate and regularity in Parkinson's disease', *Journal of the Neurological Sciences*, 310 (1–2): 231–236.

[15] Cleary, R.A., Poliakoff, E., Galpin, A., Dick, J.P.R. and Holler, J. (2011) 'An investigation of co-speech gesture production during action description in Parkinson's disease', *Parkinsonism & Related Disorders*, 17 (10): 753–756.

[16] Smith, M.C., Smith, M.K. and Ellgring, H. (1996) 'Spontaneous and posed facial expression in Parkinson's disease', *Journal of the International Neuropsychological Society*, 2 (5): 383–391.

[17] Dirnberger, G. and Jahanshahi, M. (2013) 'Executive dysfunction in Parkinson's disease: A review', *Journal of Neuropsychology*, 7 (2): 193–224.

[18] Dick, J., Fredrick, J., Man, G., Huber, J.E. and Lee, J. (2018) 'Sentence production in Parkinson's disease', *Clinical Linguistics & Phonetics*, 32 (9): 804–822.

[19] Lieberman, P., Friedman, J. and Feldman, L.S. (1990) 'Syntax comprehension deficits in Parkinson's disease', *Journal of Nervous and Mental Disease*, 178 (6): 360–365.

[20] Cousins, K.A.Q. and Grossman, M. (2017) 'Evidence of semantic processing impairments in behavioural variant frontotemporal dementia and Parkinson's disease', *Current Opinion in Neurology*, 30 (6): 617–622.

[21] Fernandino, L., Conant, L.L., Binder, J.R., Blindauer, K., Hiner, B., Spangler, K. and Desai, R.H. (2013) 'Parkinson's disease disrupts both automatic and controlled processing of action verbs', *Brain and Language*, 127 (1): 65–74.

[22] Boulenger, V., Mechtouff, L., Thobois, S., Broussolle, E., Jeannerod, M. and Nazir, T.A. (2008) 'Word processing in Parkinson's disease is impaired for action verbs but not for concrete nouns', *Neuropsychologia*, 46 (2): 743–756.

[23] Tombaugh, T.N., Kozak, J. and Rees, L. (1999) 'Normative data stratified by age and education for two measures of verbal fluency: FAS and animal naming', *Archives of Clinical Neuropsychology*, 14 (2): 167–177.

[24] Rosenthal, L.S., Salnikova, Y.A., Pontone, G.M., Pantelyat, A., Mills, K.A., Dorsey, E.R., Wang, J., Wu, S.S. and Mari, Z. (2017) 'Changes in verbal fluency in Parkinson's disease', *Movement Disorders*, 4 (1): 84–89.

[25] Deck, B.L., Rick, J., Xie, S.X., Chen-Plotkin, A., Duda, J.E., Morley, J.F., Chahine, L.M., Dahodwala, N., Trojanowski, J.Q. and Weintraub, D. (2017) 'Statins and cognition in Parkinson's disease', *Journal of Parkinson's Disease*, 7 (4): 661–667.

[26] Obeso, I., Casabona, E., Bringas, M.L., Álvarez, L. and Jahanshahi, M. (2012) 'Semantic and phonemic verbal fluency in Parkinson's disease: Influence of clinical and demographic variables', *Behavioural Neurology*, 25 (2): 111–118.

[27] Holtgraves, T. and McNamara, P. (2010) 'Pragmatic comprehension deficit in Parkinson's disease', *Journal of Clinical and Experimental Neuropsychology*, 32 (4): 388–397.

[28] Bora, E., Walterfang, M. and Velakoulis, D. (2015) 'Theory of mind in Parkinson's disease: A meta-analysis', *Behavioural Brain Research*, 292: 515–520.

[29] Monetta, L., Grindrod, C.M. and Pell, M.D. (2009) 'Irony comprehension and theory of mind deficits in patients with Parkinson's disease', *Cortex*, 45 (8): 972–981.

[30] Ellis, C., Crosson, B., Gonzalez Rothi, L.J., Okun, M.S. and Rosenbek, J.C. (2015) 'Narrative discourse cohesion in early stage Parkinson's disease', *Journal of Parkinson's Disease*, 5: 403–411. DOI:10.3233/JPD-140476.

[31] Kensinger, E.A., Shearer, D.K., Locascio, J.J., Growdon, J.H. and Corkin, S. (2003). 'Working memory in mild Alzheimer's disease and early Parkinson's disease', *Neuropsychology*, 17 (2): 230–239.

[32] Grogan, J.P., Knight, L.E., Smith, L., Izagirre, N.I., Howat, A., Knight, B.E., Bickerton, A., Isotalus, H.K. and Coulthard, E.J. (2018) 'Effects of Parkinson's disease and dopamine on digit span measures of working memory', *Psychopharmacology*, 235: 3443–3450.

[33] Montemurro, S., Mondini, S., Signorini, M., Marchetto, A., Bambini, V. and Arcara, G. (2019) 'Pragmatic language disorder in Parkinson's disease and the potential effect of cognitive reserve', *Frontiers in Psychology*, 10: 1220. doi:10.3389/fpsyg.2019.01220.

[34] Monetta, L. and Pell, M.D. (2007) 'Effects of verbal working memory deficits on metaphor comprehension in patients with Parkinson's disease', *Brain and Language*, 101 (1): 80–89.

[35] Murray, L.L. and Rutledge, S. (2014) 'Reading comprehension in Parkinson's disease', *American Journal of Speech-Language Pathology*, 23 (2): S246–S258.

CASE STUDY 7

Motor Neurone Disease

KEY FACTS AND FIGURES:

- Motor neurone disease (MND) is a progressive, neurodegenerative disease that is characterised by loss of upper motor neurons and lower motor neurons in the brain and spinal cord. The condition is also known as amyotrophic lateral sclerosis (ALS).
- The prevalence of MND is approximately six cases per 100,000. The incidence is approximately 1–2.6 cases per 100,000 persons annually.[1] MND is more common in men than in women, with a male: female sex ratio of 1.5:1.[2] The male: female sex ratio varies with age: 2.26:1 (20–49 years); 1.41:1 (50–84 years); and 1.88:1 (>85 years).[3]
- Average age of onset in MND is 58–60 years, and average survival from onset to death is 3–4 years.[1] In one clinical sample of 769 patients, long-term survival (>10 years) was associated with significantly younger onset of disease symptoms and a predominance of upper motor neuron signs at presentation.[4]
- Most cases of MND (90–95%) are sporadic and are thought to involve genetic susceptibility to environmental risk factors. The remaining 5–10% are hereditary (familial MND) and are associated with monogenic mutations in over 30 genes.[1] No replicable, definitive environmental factors have yet been identified. Factors that appear to increase the risk of MND include smoking (women), fractures (particularly in the five years before symptom onset), head/neck trauma and occupational exposure to lead and solvents/chemicals.[5–7]

DOI: 10.4324/9781003153559-8

- A wide range of motor and nonmotor symptoms occur in MND. Poor gait, balance and postural control are common in MND and result in frequent falls. Nonmotor symptoms include neuropsychiatric problems (e.g. depression, anxiety), autonomic disorders (e.g. urinary incontinence), gastrointestinal symptoms (e.g. dysphagia), and vascular problems (e.g. high cholesterol).
- Speech and language problems are common in MND. In one clinical sample, speech deteriorated to the point of requiring augmentative and alternative communication in 60% of participants.[8] In a sample of 51 patients with ALS, language impairment was found in 43%.[9]

Background

Herbert (not his real name) is 75;8 years old. He is married and has three daughters, two of whom live locally. Herbert retired in 2009 when he was 65 years old. Prior to retirement, he had worked as a self-employed financial adviser since July 1998. Herbert qualified as a chartered accountant in 1963. He worked as an accountant in industry before moving into general management and working for a textile manufacturing company. Herbert experienced a period of considerable stress at work in 1997 and 1998 and lost his job in May 1998. He was diagnosed with MND in November 2001. In November 2004, he was assessed by a consultant neurologist at a specialist motor nerve clinic in London. At that stage, Herbert was 60 years old and was very fit, often cycling 60 miles or more at weekends. He was taking riluzole 50 mg twice daily without side effects. Herbert was diagnosed as having a variant of MND called **flail arm syndrome**. Although his arms were compromised, he had no **bulbar symptoms** and, apart from some cramp and muscle twitching, his legs were normal. There was nothing to suggest familial MND. Later, in October 2014, Herbert underwent gene panel testing, in which 56 genes associated with different types of inherited neuropathy were tested. No abnormality was detected. Herbert's older brother developed **Parkinson's disease** in his seventies and is now 84 years old.

The detailed neurological examination that was conducted in November 2004 revealed mainly proximal wasting in Herbert's arms although there was also a little wasting in the intrinsic hand muscles (more on the left than the right). There were widespread **fasciculations** in the arms. Tone was normal. There was moderate arm weakness proximally and in the intrinsic hand muscles (again more marked on the left than the right). There were no tendon reflexes in the arms. Sensation was normal. There were occasional fasciculations in the legs, but tone and power were normal. The right knee jerk was abnormally brisk, and the right **adductor jerk** was brisk with a hint of crossing. The ankle jerks were normal, and the plantar responses were flexor. No abnormalities of the **cranial nerves** were found. The neurologist reported good diaphragmatic function with a forced **vital capacity** of 4.5 L (100% of predicted). Herbert was assessed to have a reasonably good **prognosis**, with no major difficulties expected with respiratory muscle weakness for several years at least. He was predicted to have a survival time of around 10 years. This time period has been well exceeded.

Prior to diagnosis in 2001, Herbert noticed several unusual signs. In about 1998, he began to get discomfort in his legs during and after cycling. In late 1999, he noticed twitching in the muscles of both arms. He visited a chiropractor on five occasions between December 2000 and February 2001. In early 2000, he noticed definite weakness in the left upper arm which was followed by weakness in the right upper arm. This was particularly noticeable when he tried to do press-ups. In August 2001, Herbert saw a rheumatologist who referred him to a neurologist. The neurologist diagnosed Herbert with MND. A series of investigations, including nerve conduction tests (February 2002), **lumbar puncture** (April 2002) and three MRI scans conducted between October 2002 and April 2004, confirmed the diagnosis.

Herbert's condition has progressed slowly since diagnosis. He first started using a wheelchair in 2010. He now has no movement of his arms and legs apart from some limited movement of his right middle finger which he can use to operate an alarm system. He sees his neurologist approximately once a year. Herbert has had no speech and language therapy but has received some physiotherapy and considerable occupational therapy. Carers visit each day to assist Herbert's wife in providing him with personal care. Herbert has been hospitalised for heart and urinary problems but for nothing directly related to his MND. He has had occasional bouts of gout in the past. Herbert uses an in-dwelling catheter. He has medical appointments in podiatry and to regularly change his catheter.

Clinical Symptoms

Herbert has no mobility and uses a wheelchair all the time. He does not report any sensory symptoms. He states that there is "nothing unusual" with his **memory**, concentration, **planning** and **attention** "for someone of my age". His immobility has given rise to some digestive problems, constipation and fluid retention. Herbert has neck weakness that necessitates care when swallowing. He can experience frustration which leads to mild **depression**, but this is "not a big issue". He reports no impact of MND on either his speech or language.

Daily Activities

Herbert reports that all daily activities are compromised as a result of his MND. For the last 10 years of work, Herbert had MND. During this time, driving became increasingly difficult, especially when he had to raise his arms to the steering wheel after changing gears. He also found it difficult to lift down files at work. As his walking became affected, he bought a wheelchair that was initially used only when he went outside. However, he began to have falls and started to use the wheelchair in the house as well. Herbert and his wife enjoyed walking with friends which was affected as his mobility became impaired. Herbert reports that he and his wife were "not great holiday people" even before the onset of MND. Although they do not travel now, they have undertaken several trips in the past, including a river cruise, a trip to Tuscany for Herbert's 50th birthday and summer holidays in his brother's cottage. Herbert became heavily involved in a local charity which was established in 2008 with the purpose of restoring an old church building and converting it into an arts and heritage centre. He became a trustee and honorary treasurer until 2017 when he was no longer able to cope with the physical demands of these roles. Today, he enjoys attending concerts and other events in the centre, especially classical and sacred choral music.

Herbert enjoys reading but can no longer use a Kindle. Instead, he listens to audio books. He likes a wide range of authors and subjects, both fiction and non-fiction. Herbert can type email messages using Grid Pad and an Eye Gaze camera attached to his wheelchair. With the use of this technology, his eyes can track the keys on an ordinary keyboard without having to move his head or neck. Sometimes, for ease and convenience, his wife types emails for him. Herbert watches some TV. His interests include comedy, travel and farming programmes, and watching rugby. He also likes to keep abreast of politics. Herbert is dependent on his wife and carers for all aspects of his personal care.

Medication

Herbert does not take medication related to his MND. On the advice of his neurologist, he stopped taking riluzole several years ago. He has some heart, blood pressure and digestive problems that are controlled by medication. There are no side effects of these drugs.

Communication

Relative to his other difficulties, Herbert's communication skills are an area of strength. As described above, Herbert's ability to read and write are compromised as a result of his motor disability. He is no longer able to hold a book and turn its pages, use a pen to write, or type using a keyboard. Herbert's severe motor disability also prevents him using **gesture** during communication. However, in many other respects he is a very competent communicator who can participate fully in conversation. His speech production is 100% intelligible. Herbert produces well-formed utterances and understands the utterances of others. He is also highly motivated to communicate and contributes utterances as well as responds to the utterances of his communication partners. Herbert makes effective use of facial expression during communication. Communication is not impaired by hearing loss or visual impairment.

The author visited Herbert at home on 7 February 2020. His wife was present during the visit. Herbert was in his wheelchair in the living room and the entire session was conducted in this location. The author sat in an armchair next to Herbert. Herbert's wife sat for part of the session but moved between the living room and kitchen to undertake various tasks. Herbert was positioned with the large living room window behind him to give him as much daylight as possible for the tasks. When he had to examine pictures, a stand was placed on the table at the front of his wheelchair and positioned to avoid glare from sunlight. Herbert was cooperative and responsive throughout the session. He did not fatigue and did not require a break between tasks.

Herbert's speech production is fully intelligible. He can articulate speech sounds and has normal **resonance** and **voice quality**. His respiratory support for speech, vocal volume, **intonation** and stress are also in the normal range. Herbert has good speech **fluency** and speaks at a normal rate. There was no evidence of **dysarthria** or **apraxia of speech**. Herbert does not have a phonological impairment.

There is evidence of impairments in expressive and receptive language in MND. In one study of 34 participants with MND, accuracy on a range of language domains varied, but was generally in excess of 83%: **confrontation naming** (83%); single-word repetition (89%); semantic association (91%); word comprehension (92%); and sentence comprehension (96%).[10] Spelling is also impaired in MND.[11,12] Herbert's expressive language is well structured. He used a wide range of inflectional and derivational morphemes during the session, several of which are illustrated below:

Inflectional morphemes: retir<u>ed</u>; sister<u>s</u>; happi<u>est</u>; break<u>s</u>; horse<u>'s</u> head; draw<u>ing</u>

Derivational morphemes:

Prefixes: <u>un</u>comfortable; <u>in</u>appropriate; <u>down</u>load
Suffixes: advis<u>er</u>; manufactur<u>ing</u>; financ<u>ial</u>; sugges<u>tion</u>; activ<u>ity</u>; manage<u>ment</u>; ill<u>ness</u>

There is evidence of impaired auditory comprehension of complex sentences in MND.[12,13] Deficits in grammatical expression that are independent of motor disorder are also reported.[14] However, Herbert was also able to produce and understand utterances with complex **syntax**. He was able to comprehend a range of constructions such as the interrogative **subordinate clause** and the **relative clause** in the utterances below:

Interrogative subordinate clause:

Can you tell me <u>what type of work you were doing before you retired</u>?

Relative clause:

> Do you have any interests and hobbies <u>that you pursue in your free time</u>?

Herbert displayed intact expressive syntax. He used several complex grammatical structures, including **passive voice** constructions and *that*-clauses:

Passive voice construction:

> "Ended up working for a textile manufacturing company which <u>was ultimately taken over by a PLC based in Scotland</u>"

That-clause:

> I didn't explain to you <u>that ah (.) I was born in XXX</u>

Herbert displayed intact naming of nouns. He named 17 of 18 words correctly during the confrontation naming task. The only stimulus item that posed difficulty for him was *ostrich* which he named 'turkey'. However, following presentation of the **semantic cue** below, Herbert was able to name the item correctly:

> it's a very large bird, we can eat this bird, we don't do it often, but people do eat the meat of this bird, lays very large eggs and can run extremely fast

There is evidence that the naming of verbs is more impaired than the naming of nouns in MND,[15] and also that action verbs where the body is the **agent** of an action are more impaired than action verbs where the body is the theme.[16] Herbert was able to produce and understand a range of verbs without difficulty. He made extensive use of action verbs like *stroking, walking* and *giving*, where the body is the agent of an action. Action verbs in MND and other **neurodegenerative disorders** (e.g. **Parkinson's disease**) are impaired on account of degradation of the semantic representation of action related to motor dysfunction.

Herbert did not report, or display any evidence of, word-finding difficulties in conversation. However, he did find it difficult to generate animal names during a semantic (category) fluency task. He produced 13 animal names in 60 seconds. This score was not only lower than normative values for healthy individuals without neurodegenerative disorders,[17-19] but was also lower than normative values for people with MND.[17] Although Herbert's confrontation naming performance showed that he could access and retrieve words from his mental lexicon in response to visual stimuli, the spontaneous generation needed to execute a **semantic fluency** task was clearly an additional cognitive challenge for him. Phonemic (letter) fluency, however, was an area of strength for Herbert.

He produced 13 words beginning with the letter F in 60 seconds. This is slightly above normative values for individuals with MND,[10,17,20] and is consistent with the **phonemic fluency** performance of healthy participants without neurodegenerative disorders.[17,18] Herbert's **letter fluency** score suggests his **executive function** skills are intact.

Herbert displayed strengths in his use of complex meaning relations. He was able to conjoin **clauses** according to conceptual relations such as *time, reason, consequence* and *condition*:

> before I retired, I was ah a financial adviser
>
> *(time)*

> there was huge stress 'cause I was starting from a base of zero
>
> *(reason)*

> the pension scheme … went bust as well so that added to my problems
>
> *(consequence)*

> provided I managed to keep them on the steering wheel, I was okay
>
> *(condition)*

Herbert also used a range of semantic or participant roles to characterise entities in a situation. They included *source, goal, patient, theme* and *location*, as illustrated by these utterances:

> from the balcony [SOURCE] a pot plant [PATIENT] falls through and hits him on the head [GOAL]
> it [THEME] sat out there in the sunroom [LOCATION]

Herbert displayed many intact pragmatic language and **discourse** skills. He was able to contribute relevant, informative utterances to conversation. Herbert was aware of the need to be maximally informative in conversation. This expectation is acknowledged in the following utterance where he explicitly signals through use of the hedge *to cut a long story short* that he is trying to avoid conveying too much information:

> and em (1.33) long story short the PLC that took over the company I'd been with for twenty (.) six years (1.08) didn't have a good relationship and ah business was going badly

Herbert made effective use of **idioms** and **hyperbole** in his expressive language. The idioms in these utterances convey the failing status of the company Herbert worked for, Herbert's unwillingness to consider forms of employment other than senior management positions and an author's description of the impact of spinal injury on her life:

> both that company and the company that I'd been with were <u>on the skids</u> initially I had <u>the blinkers on</u>
> she doesn't eh (1.04) <u>miss the mark</u>, does she?

Herbert used hyperbole when describing the amount of reading he had undertaken since retirement:

> what else have I read oh (1.22) <u>miles and miles of stuff</u>

Herbert was skilled at monitoring and correcting his verbal output. In the following utterance, he undertakes self-initiated self-repair when describing the year that he lost his job:

> I lost my job in nineteen ninety-eight eh ah nineteen ninety (1.45) xxx (*unintelligible*) (.) nineteen ninety-four actually

Herbert used a range of **deictic expressions**, including instances of spatial deixis (*here, there*) and personal deixis (*you, me*) in the utterances below:

> I was born in XXX which is another reason why we returned <u>here</u> at retirement
> it must have been very frustrating for <u>you</u> sitting <u>there</u> listening to <u>me</u>

A discourse device that is used to engage hearers and readers is **direct reported speech**. Herbert used this device in conversation when he described advice that he received from his brother-in-law to pursue self-employment:

> the suggestion was made "why don't you follow my (0.83) eh (0.88) course and ah and eh you know try your hand at doing something on your own?"

Finally, Herbert also used several linguistic devices to achieve **cohesion** between utterances. In the following examples of **lexical substitution**, *one* is a substitute for the noun 'book' in (A) and a substitute for 'question' in (B). In (B), the noun 'question' is not explicitly stated but is nevertheless understood in the prior discourse context:

A. "*Far from the Madding Crowd* is <u>one</u> that I've just read"
B. INV: do you have a holiday … that you've really enjoyed?

>   PAR: ah that's in (0.72) an interesting <u>one</u>

Another **cohesive device** used by Herbert was **anaphoric reference**. In (C), the **demonstrative pronoun** *that* refers anaphorically to 'worked for another subsidiary', while in (D) the **personal pronoun** *them* refers to 'books':

C. "and worked for another subsidiary in (.) Ayrshire (.) but <u>that</u> ah (1.36) didn't work well"
D. "I can download books and listen to <u>them</u>"

Consistent with reports in the literature,[21,22] Herbert also displayed some pragmatic language and **discourse** difficulties. On occasion, he drew mistaken **inferences** which were nonetheless plausible in context. During immediate recall of the Sam and Fred story, Herbert related that the farmers "called for help" when the story simply stated that "people from the local village arrived to help the two distressed farmers". Also, Herbert did not appear able to draw an inference about the mother's mental state during the Cookie Theft picture description task. The mother in the picture had not noticed that the sink was overflowing because she was daydreaming or distracted. However, Herbert was unaware of these mental states when he said:

don't know why she hasn't noticed that the eh (0.88) water's spilling over

MND speakers with bulbar signs have been found to have difficulty attributing mental states to characters in cartoons and narratives, a deficit related to **theory of mind** (ToM).[23] A similar ToM-related difficulty may explain Herbert's failure of mental state attribution in this case.

Herbert was able to produce detailed narratives. Occasionally, however, he omitted key information such as that the storm blew open the door of the barn in the Sam and Fred story and that Cinderella's father died, an event that is essential to understanding how Cinderella came to be at the mercy of her stepmother. Although Herbert stated that the young girl in the Cookie Theft picture description task is trying to get cookies out of the cookie jar, he omitted to mention that she was gesturing to her brother to be quiet in order to evade detection by their mother. Herbert occasionally conveyed incorrect information and non-specific information. The gentleman in the Flowerpot Incident narrative was not entering his own home ("gets close to his front door"). Also, it was the crops that were washed away by the storm in the Sam and Fred story, not the more generally characterised "results of all their hard labour". Herbert's difficulties with information are consistent with published findings. Discourse productivity (measured by MLU, total words and total utterances) is less impaired than discourse content (measured by percent correct information units and content units) during picture description in speakers with ALS without **dementia**.[24]

COMMUNICATION PROFILE:

Speech intelligibility:

- Herbert's speech production is 100% intelligible; articulation of speech sounds, resonance, breathing for speech, voice quality, intonation and stress are in the normal range; Herbert speaks with normal fluency and rate; Herbert does not have dysarthria and apraxia of speech; there is no evidence of phonological impairment.

Morphology and syntax:

- Herbert's expressive language is well formed; he uses a range of inflectional and derivational morphemes; Herbert can produce and understand utterances with complex syntax including interrogative subordinate and relative clauses and passive voice constructions.

Vocabulary and semantics:

- Herbert has a high-level vocabulary; he has no word-finding difficulties in conversation; his confrontation naming ability is intact; semantic fluency is reduced relative to healthy individuals and people with MND; Herbert can express complex meaning relations in language and is able to use a range of semantic roles.

Pragmatics:

- Herbert displays several pragmatic language skills; he uses figurative language such as idioms and hyperbole, presuppositions and deixis; he is able to fulfil conversational expectations by contributing relevant, informative utterances in conversation; Herbert can monitor his verbal output and uses repair strategies; occasionally he fails to draw inferences about the mental states of characters in scenes and narratives, although he uses mental state language.

Discourse:

- Herbert uses cohesive devices such as lexical substitution and anaphoric reference to link utterances in discourse; he can introduce direct reported speech into conversation; he sometimes omits key information in narratives and conveys incorrect and non-specific information; his use of story grammar is intact.

Cognition:

- Herbert's phonemic fluency score is superior to people with MND and consistent with that of healthy individuals, suggesting that his executive function skills are an area of strength; Herbert reports intact memory and other cognitive skills for someone of his years; his extensive use of pauses in discourse suggest that he requires more time for the planning of his utterances.

Suggestions for Further Reading

(1) Pinto-Grau, M., Hardiman, O. and Pender, N. (2018) 'The study of language in the amyotrophic lateral sclerosis – frontotemporal spectrum disorder: A systematic review of findings and new perspectives', *Neuropsychology Review*, 28 (2): 251–268.

   This systematic review characterises the profile of language dysfunction in ALS. Deficits in word retrieval, syntactic and grammatical processing and spelling are reported, although the authors acknowledge that understanding of the ALS language profile is limited by studies using small clinical samples.

(2) Roberts-South, A., Findlater, K., Strong, M.J. and Orange, J.B. (2012) 'Longitudinal changes in discourse production in amyotrophic lateral sclerosis', *Seminars in Speech and Language*, 33 (1): 79–94.

   While language in general has received little investigation in ALS, the area of discourse has been particularly neglected. This study uses a picture description task to examine discourse production in ALS, and charts the decline of discourse skills (specifically, discourse content) with disease progression.

(3) Tomik, B. and Guiloff, R.J. (2010) 'Dysarthria in amyotrophic lateral sclerosis: A review', *Amyotrophic Lateral Sclerosis*, 11 (1-2): 4–15.

   Traditionally, the speech disorder in ALS is the reason given for the involvement of speech-language pathologists in the care of people with ALS. With growing recognition of the role of nonmotor symptoms in ALS, language and cognitive impairments are now addressed alongside speech disorder. This review examines the clinical features, differential diagnosis and pathophysiology of dysarthria in ALS as well as the management of this speech disorder.

Questions

(1) Herbert is a skilled narrator who produced for the most part informative, well-structured narratives during the session. One such narrative is the Cinderella story which is presented in full below. Examine this narrative and then answer the questions below it:

> poor unfortunate Cinderella (0.70) ah (1.17) she lost her mother and ah her father was looking after her (1.40) and her father decided to get married again (1.49) and em (1.84) Cinderella went to live (0.95) with the father and the stepmother and two stepdaughters (2.01) and she was brought into the house instead of being treated like a proper daughter (0.74) she was very (0.77) badly treated and made to do all the menial tasks about the house (1.12) em (2.31) but she also looked after the animals (1.07) and she ah found the animals all loved her (0.93) with the exception of one rather nasty (0.70) cat … the king of the kingdom

who's getting old and ah (1.07) worried about succession (1.26) and gets his (1.21) ah (2.57) whatever you would call him what's he called chief assistant or representative or whatever (1.42) em (1.63) to ah (1.12) organise a ball (1.61) and invite all the eligible (0.72) young ladies eh to come to the ball to see if they can find a suitable wife ah for his son (1.07) so the ball was organised and ah (1.26) em (0.64) stepmother and her daughters (1.21) are all invited to the ball (1.46) the stepmother's very anxious that one of her (.) own daughters em is chosen (1.00) eh but Cinderella is included as well but she's (.) dressed up in (1.34) inappropriate (0.65) em (0.70) attire … she finds herself very unhappily sitting on the steps outside and ah (1.10) this old lady comes and chats to her (0.77) and ah (2.91) the old lady listens to her story (1.11) and (1.43) suddenly becomes her (1.37) ah fairy godmother (2.62) and (1.39) ah uses her own magic charms to (1.37) am converted the pumpkin into a royal carriage and the mice into (0.88) the horses that (.) transport (1.00) Cinderella ump eh to the ball (0.94) and (0.94) she is all beautifully dressed (0.67) magic clothes I guess as well (0.88) including two wonderful magic slippers (1.42) em (2.97) and the one (1.34) criterion is that (0.73) all of this magic that she's enjoying at the ball eh (0.63) ends at midnight and she must be home before midnight (1.98) but she enjoys it all so much that she loses (1.10) ah (0.80) sense of time and by midnight it's too late she hasn't got back to the house (0.93) and ah (0.85) she races down the steps outside and one of the slippers falls off (1.81) ah (1.42) but suddenly she's (.) transported back into her rags (1.57) and (.) back into the house again back into (0.70) all the (1.18) em old way of life (0.67) but she has retained one slipper (1.60) ah (1.08) in the meantime the prince (1.50) em remembers this girl (1.20) and (0.88) has the other slipper and (1.03) the king sends his (0.75) uh emissary whatever out to try and find the (1.48) beautiful ump eh person girl that (1.18) eh the slipper will fit (1.41) and (1.65) ultimately (0.84) finds Cinderella where the slipper fits perfectly she's brought to the (1.29) palace meets the prince fall in love are married (1.18) and (0.94) happy end

(a) Herbert retains an extensive vocabulary. Along with high-frequency words such as *house* and *lady*, he uses several low-frequency words. Identify *four* such words in his narrative.

(b) Herbert is skilled at attributing mental states to the minds of the protagonists in this narrative. Identify *three* verbs used by Herbert to attribute mental states to the characters in the story. What cognitive capacity underlies Herbert's use of these verbs?

(c) At one point during his narration, Herbert engages in metalinguistic discourse. Where does this occur in the narrative?

(d) Herbert's narrative is littered with many pauses, a substantial number of which are over one second in duration. Why might these pauses occur?

(e) It was described in the main text how Herbert neglected to mention that Cinderella's father died. Herbert also omits another important event in the story. What is this event?

(2) Presupposition is a pragmatic language skill. Herbert used several linguistic expressions that trigger presuppositions. Some of these expressions are underlined in the utterances below. Match each of these expressions to one of the following terms in italics. What is the presupposition triggered by each of these expressions? *factive verb – temporal clause – implicative verb – change-of-state verb – iterative*

(a) "they <u>managed</u> to do by nightfall"
(b) "her father decided to get married <u>again</u>"
(c) "<u>before</u> I retired, I was ah a financial advisor"
(d) "don't <u>know</u> why she hasn't noticed that the eh water's spilling over"
(e) "and then <u>began</u> to find it very difficult to secure such a job"

(3) Herbert produced the following description of the Cookie Theft picture from the Boston Diagnostic Aphasia Examination.[25] Examine his description and then answer the questions below:

> okay well I see mum doing the dishes (1.22) ah she doesn't seem to notice that the tap's still running and it's (.) water's pouring out over the edge on to the floor em (1.63) it looks like her son and daughter are trying to (0.70) eh get cookies out of the cookie jar (0.70) but the son's on top of the stool which is falling over there's going to be a (.) an accident very soon

(a) Herbert undertakes self-initiated self-repair during his description. Where does this occur?

(b) Herbert's lexical abilities are an area of strength. If his lexical skills were impaired, what words might he use in place of *mum, son* and *daughter*?

(c) It was described in the main text how Herbert failed to draw an inference about the mother's mental state. This inference would explain why the mother had not turned off the tap. Herbert's description also overlooks other mental states of the actors in the picture. What are these mental states?

(d) There are several timed pauses in Herbert's description. Describe their significance.

(e) Herbert uses anaphoric reference to achieve cohesion between utterances at one point in this description. Where does it occur?

Answers

(1) (a) succession; attire; criterion; emissary
   (b) "the stepmother's very <u>anxious</u>"; "her father <u>decided</u> to get married again"; "the prince <u>remembers</u> this girl"; cognitive capacity = theory of mind
   (c) metalinguistic discourse: "and gets his (1.21) ah (2.57) <u>whatever you would call him what's he called chief assistant or representative or whatever</u>"
   (d) The pauses in Herbert's narrative provide him with additional time for information processing. This gives Herbert the time he needs to plan his utterances, from deciding what information needs to be communicated to formulating the linguistic utterances that convey this information.
   (e) Herbert does not state that Cinderella met the prince at the ball. In fact, he relates that Cinderella met the prince for the first time at the very end of the narrative.
(2) (a) implicative verb – they tried to do X by nightfall
   (b) iterative – her father was married before
   (c) temporal clause – Herbert retired
   (d) factive verb – she hasn't noticed the water's spilling over
   (e) change-of-state verb – Herbert had previously not found it difficult to secure such a job
(3) (a) self-initiated self-repair: "it's (.) water's pouring out over the edge"
   (b) If Herbert had impaired lexical abilities, he might use the more general words *woman, boy* and *girl* in place of the more specific words *mother, son* and *daughter*, respectively.
   (c) The boy and girl in the picture are engaged in an act of deception. They *want* to take the cookies from the jar, but they *know* that their mother will not permit them to have the cookies. So, they act surreptitiously behind her back in the *knowledge* that their mother is *daydreaming* and will not *realise* what is happening. The words in italics are the mental states that can be attributed to the children's minds and to the mind of their mother. Herbert's description does not address any of these states.
   (d) With one exception, Herbert's timed pauses occur at grammatical boundaries. The location of these pauses suggests that Herbert needs additional time to plan and encode his utterances.
   (e) anaphoric reference: "I see <u>mum</u> doing the dishes (1.22) ah <u>she</u> doesn't seem to notice …"

References

[1] Talbott, E.O., Malek, A.M. and Lacomis, D. (2016) 'The epidemiology of amyotrophic lateral sclerosis', in C. Rosano, M.A. Ikram and M. Ganguli (eds), *Handbook of Clinical Neurology, Volume 138: Neuroepidemiology*. Elsevier, 225–238.
[2] Wijesekera, L.C. and Leigh, P.N. (2009) 'Amyotrophic lateral sclerosis', *Orphanet Journal of Rare Diseases*, 4:3. doi: 10.1186/1750-1172-4-3.

[3] Ahmadzai, P., Kab, S., Vlaar, T., Artaud, F., Carcaillon-Bentata, L., Canonico, M., Moisan, F. and Elbaz, A. (2018) 'Age-dependent sex ratios of motor neuron disease: French nationwide study and meta-analysis', *Neurology*, 90 (18): e1588–e1595.

[4] Turner, M.R., Parton, M.J., Shaw, C.E., Leigh, P.N. and Al-Chalabi, A. (2003) 'Prolonged survival in motor neuron disease: A descriptive study of the King's database 1990–2002', *Journal of Neurology Neurosurgery & Psychiatry*, 74 (7): 995–997.

[5] Doyle, P., Brown, A., Beral, V., Reeves, G. and Green, J. (2012) 'Incidence of and risk factors for motor neurone disease in UK women: A prospective study', *BMC Neurology*, 12: 25. doi: 10.1186/1471-2377-12-25.

[6] Chancellor, A.M., Slattery, J.M., Fraser, H. and Warlow, C.P. (1993) 'Risk factors for motor neuron disease: A case-control study based on patients from the Scottish Motor Neuron Disease Register', *Journal of Neurology, Neurosurgery & Psychiatry*, 56 (11): 1200–1206.

[7] Cui, F., Liu, M., Chen, Y., Huang, X., Cui, L., Fan, D., Pu, C., Lu, J., Zhou, D., Zhang, C., Yan, C., Li, C., Ding, X., Liu, Y., Li, X., Jiang, Y., Zhang, J., Shang, H., Yao, X., Ding, Y., Niu, Q. and Wang, L. (2014) 'Epidemiological characteristics of motor neuron disease in Chinese patients', *Acta Neurologica Scandinavica*, 130 (2): 111–117.

[8] Makkonen, T., Ruottinen, H., Puhto, R., Helminen, M. and Palmio, J. (2018) 'Speech deterioration in amyotrophic lateral sclerosis (ALS) after manifestation of bulbar symptoms', *International Journal of Language & Communication Disorders*, 53 (2): 385–392.

[9] Taylor, L.J., Brown, R.G., Tsermentseli, S., Al-Chalabi, A., Shaw, C.E., Ellis, C.M., Leigh, P.N. and Goldstein, L.H. (2013) 'Is language impairment more common than executive dysfunction in amyotrophic lateral sclerosis?', *Journal of Neurology, Neurosurgery, and Psychiatry*, 84 (5): 494–498.

[10] Long, Z., Irish, M., Piguet, O., Kiernan, M.C., Hodges, J.R. and Burrell, J.R. (2019) 'Clinical and neuroimaging investigations of language disturbance in frontotemporal dementia-motor neuron disease patients', *Journal of Neurology*, 266: 921–933.

[11] Pinto-Grau, M., Hardiman, O. and Pender, N. (2018) 'The study of language in the amyotrophic lateral sclerosis-frontotemporal spectrum disorder: A systematic review of findings and new perspectives', *Neuropsychology Review*, 28 (2): 251–268.

[12] Cobble, M. (1998) 'Language impairment in motor neurone disease', *Journal of the Neurological Sciences*, 160 (Suppl 1): S47–S52.

[13] Tsermentseli, S., Leigh, P.N., Taylor, L.J., Radunovic, A., Catani, M. and Goldstein, L.H. (2015) 'Syntactic processing as a marker for cognitive impairment in amyotrophic lateral sclerosis', *Amyotrophic Lateral Sclerosis & Frontotemporal Degeneration*, 17 (1–2): 69–76.

[14] Ash, S., Olm, C., McMillan, C.T., Boller, A., Irwin, D.J., McCluskey, L., Elman, L. and Grossman, M. (2015) 'Deficits in sentence expression in amyotrophic lateral sclerosis', *Amyotrophic Lateral Sclerosis & Frontotemporal Degeneration*, 16 (1–2): 31–39.

[15] Bak, T.H. and Hodges, J.R. (2004) 'The effects of motor neurone disease on language: Further evidence', *Brain and Language*, 89: 354–361.

[16] Cousins, K.A.Q., Ash, S. and Grossman, M. (2018) 'Production of verbs related to body movement in amyotrophic lateral sclerosis (ALS) and Parkinson's disease (PD)', *Cortex*, 100: 127–139.

[17] Lepow, L., Van Sweringen, J., Strutt, A.M., Jawaid, A., MacAdam, C., Harati, Y., Schulz, P.E. and York, M.K. (2010) 'Frontal and temporal lobe involvement on verbal fluency measures in amyotrophic lateral sclerosis', *Journal of Clinical and Experimental Neuropsychology*, 32 (9): 913–922.

[18] Tombaugh, T.N., Kozak, J. and Rees, L. (1999) 'Normative data stratified by age and education for two measures of verbal fluency: FAS and animal naming', *Archives of Clinical Neuropsychology*, 14 (2): 167–177.

[19] Acevedo, A., Loewenstein, D.A., Barker, W.W., Harwood, D.G., Luis, C., Bravo, M., Hurwitz, D.A., Aguero, H., Greenfield, L. and Duara, R. (2000) 'Category fluency test: Normative data for English- and Spanish-speaking elderly', *Journal of the International Neuropsychological Society*, 6: 760–769.

[20] Quinn, C., Elman, L., McCluskey, L., Hoskins, K., Karam, C., Woo, J.H., Poptani, H., Wang, S., Chawla, S., Kasner, S.E. and Grossman, M. (2012) 'Frontal lobe abnormalities on MRS correlate with poor letter fluency in ALS', *Neurology*, 79 (6): 583–588.

[21] Bambini, V., Arcara, G., Martinelli, I., Bernini, S., Alvisi, E., Moro, A., Cappa, S.F. and Ceroni, M. (2016) 'Communication and pragmatic breakdowns in amyotrophic lateral sclerosis patients', *Brain & Language*, 153–154: 1–12.

[22] Bloch, S., Saldert, C. and Ferm, U. (2015) 'Problematic topic transitions in dysarthric conversation', *International Journal of Speech-Language Pathology*, 17 (4): 373–383.

[23] Gibbons, Z.C., Snowden, J.S., Thompson, J.C., Happé, F., Richardson, A. and Neary, D. (2007) 'Inferring thought and action in motor neurone disease', *Neuropsychologia*, 45 (6): 1196–1207.

[24] Roberts-South, A., Findlater, K., Strong, M.J. and Orange, J.B. (2012) 'Longitudinal changes in discourse production in amyotrophic lateral sclerosis', *Seminars in Speech and Language*, 33 (1): 79–94.

[25] Goodglass, H., Kaplan, E. and Barresi, B. (2001) *Boston Diagnostic Aphasia Examination*, third Edition. Baltimore: Lippincott Williams & Wilkins.

CASE STUDY 8

Alcohol-Related Brain Damage

KEY FACTS AND FIGURES:

- Alcohol-related brain damage (ARBD) describes changes in brain structure and function caused by chronic alcohol consumption in the absence of well-characterised alcohol-related conditions such as Wernicke's encephalopathy (WE) and Korsakoff syndrome (KS).[1]
- Neurological dysfunction in ARBD, WE and KS is related to thiamine (vitamin B1) deficiency. In people who abuse alcohol, there is reduced dietary supply of the vitamin due to malnutrition and malabsorption. Additionally, liver damage leads to poor storage and processing of thiamine.[2]
- The prevalence of ARBD varies considerably across studies. Prevalence is reported to be 21% among homeless hostel dwellers in Glasgow.[3] The prevalence of ARBD in new and old long-stay mental hospital patients in Scotland is 9% and 5%, respectively.[4] It is estimated that 35% of those with alcohol dependence will exhibit post-mortem evidence of ARBD.[5] The more severe Wernicke-Korsakoff syndrome (WKS) occurs in 1–2% of the general population in the United States.[6] The prevalence of WKS has decreased in countries that have instituted nationwide thiamine enrichment of staple foods such as bread.[7]
- ARBD affects people in their forties and fifties, with women presenting a decade younger than men.[5] In a clinical sample of 51 patients with Wernicke's encephalopathy, 78.4% were male. The median age at diagnosis and death were 57 years and 65 years, respectively.[8]

DOI: 10.4324/9781003153559-9

- ARBD and WKS are associated with cognitive impairments (memory, visuospatial function), psychiatric and behavioural disorders (depression, apathy, agitation, aggression), and physical problems.[9,10] Confusion, ataxia, and ophthalmoplegia or nystagmus are the triad of clinical features associated with WKS, although only 16% of patients are reported to exhibit the full triad and 19% are reported to have no documented clinical signs.[11]

Background

Sammy (not his real name) is 51;7 years old. He is divorced and has a 20-year-old daughter. His daughter lives locally to him but they are estranged from each other. Sammy formerly worked as an upholsterer and owned his own upholstery business. He left school at 16 years of age. Sammy was diagnosed with ARBD in April 2019. He has a history of excessive alcohol consumption, beginning in adolescence and persisting throughout adulthood. Sammy was drinking up to 180 units per week. This has resulted in several hospital admissions to treat injuries related to falls and to supervise withdrawal from alcohol. In February 2018, Sammy was admitted to hospital for the treatment of eight broken ribs, a serious injury that was sustained in a fall down the stairs at his home. The hospital admission during which he was diagnosed with ARBD occurred between 6 April 2019 and 1 May 2019. This admission, which was an emergency, was prompted by alcohol withdrawal seizures. Sammy's first seizure occurred in his parents' home and the second one took place in the emergency department of his local hospital. Both seizures were self-limiting. During his stay in hospital, Sammy was under the care of a gastroenterologist and the hospital's Alcohol Awareness Team.

Clinical Symptoms

Sammy's admission to hospital followed a period of heavy drinking that stopped one day prior to his seizures. On admission, he was in a state of agitation and was administered 1 mg lorazepam. He made a full recovery from the seizures. He was commenced on Pabrinex, fluids and Librium (chlordiaepoxide). (Pabrinex is an injection that contains vitamins B and C that may be started in the emergency department to prevent **Wernicke's encephalopathy**. Librium is used to treat withdrawal symptoms from alcohol.) Sammy received prolonged treatment with Pabrinex as the medical staff suspected WE. He was diagnosed with hypokalaemia (low level of potassium in the blood serum) and hyponatraemia (serum sodium less than 135 mmol/L), both of which resolved. His electrocardiogram (ECG) displayed a prolonged QTc. (The clinical significance of a prolonged QTc is uncertain, as there is no consistent evidence for increased risks of total or cardiovascular mortality or of sudden death associated with prolonged QTc interval.[12]) Sammy obtained a score of 17/30 (moderate cognitive impairment) on the Montreal Cognitive Assessment (MoCA) on admission to hospital. Eleven days later, on 17 April 2019, his MoCA assessment was repeated and he scored 22/30 (**mild cognitive impairment**).

During his stay in hospital, Sammy underwent computerised tomography of his brain. There was no evidence of a focal intraparenchymal mass lesion on this unenhanced study. There was a background of bilateral cerebral and cerebellar **atrophy**. He also developed a left axillary abscess. This had been previously drained in hospital and recurred while Sammy was an inpatient. He was commenced on flucloxacillin and the site was dressed daily. He continued taking antibiotics for 10 days in total. Sammy's sister reported that he was extremely ill as an inpatient. He became incontinent, very weak and was confused. She said he repeated himself to excess and at one stage thought that his deceased brother had come to visit him. Sammy's difficulties with alcohol consumption were evident while he was in hospital. Bottles of whisky and beer were found in his room by the occupational therapist and nursing staff. He did not appear to understand how inappropriate this was in a hospital setting and when he was being treated for detoxification. Sammy left the ward multiple times a day supposedly to smoke cigarettes, but there was a strong suspicion among ward staff that this was to drink alcohol. Sammy claimed that he did not realise that it was wrong to do this in hospital. He was visited multiple times during his admission by substance misuse liaison staff. He was also followed up by them on discharge.

Sammy was assessed by the medical team as having capacity and as medically fit for discharge. He was discharged from hospital to his parents' home where he received help with practical activities of daily living and medication. On discharge from hospital, Sammy was still taking flucloxacillin. He was commenced on thiamine and vitamin B compound strong tablets. He was also taking paracetamol and using Tears Naturale for dry eyes. An outpatient ultrasound scan of his liver was arranged because of deranged liver function tests (GAMMA GT scores in excess of 500) and suspicion of **cirrhosis**. He was advised not to drive.

Daily Activities

Prior to his most recent hospital stay, Sammy struggled with all activities of daily living. His work duties were compromised by extended periods of inebriation. He was often unable to shop for food and cook regular meals. As a result, he experienced poor nutrition. He had a loss of appetite and was frequently unable to finish a meal. During periods of heavy drinking, Sammy did not attend to personal hygiene. He relied on the assistance of a friend to maintain the cleanliness of his house. Sammy had financial difficulties and was frequently behind in the payment of bills. His social relationships were also negatively affected by his drinking. Membership of his local golf club was cancelled after he had several confrontational encounters with other members and staff. His housemate found alternative accommodation following a series of arguments with Sammy. Sammy was unable to find another tenant to share the rent and eventually had to leave the property.

After discharge from hospital, Sammy's sister became directly involved in his care. She found him rented accommodation and furnished it for him. Sammy now lives within walking distance of his parents' house and the home of another brother. Sammy's sister also took charge of his finances. She applied for social security benefits on Sammy's behalf as he was no longer able to work. Sammy receives access to the local food bank. His sister also arranged for carers to visit him twice daily to check on compliance with medication. Sammy is also under the supervision of an addiction support worker. He was able to abstain from alcohol immediately after discharge and while he was staying with his parents. However, he has been unable to maintain abstinence while living independently. Recently, the relationship with his sister has deteriorated around financial issues. She is no longer assisting him with daily activities or managing his finances for him.

Medication

Sammy is taking two vitamin B compound strong tablets three times a day. He is also taking one thiamine 100 mg tablet three times a day. Carers visit Sammy twice a day to ensure that he is taking his medication as directed.

Communication

The author visited Sammy at his home in the afternoon of 17 August 2019. He was 3.5 months post-discharge and had just moved into his new house. His sister had managed to furnish most rooms in the house although some further work was still required. Sammy was physically well and had attended the outpatient appointment for the ultrasound scan of his liver the day before. He had found this a very stressful experience as he and his mother struggled to find the health facility where the procedure was performed. Sammy spoke in a positive way about plans for his future. He showed the author around the outside of his house where there were two sheds. He intended to upgrade these sheds and use them to resume his upholstery work. He also wanted to join the local golf club and had already taken out gym membership. He was still smoking and had occasionally lapsed and consumed alcohol. He was talkative and cooperative throughout the test session. He requested a break in the audio-recording so that he could go outside to have a cigarette.

Sammy had normal speech production skills. There was no **dysarthria** or **apraxia of speech**. His **articulation** of speech sounds was intact. He had normal **resonance** and breath support for speech and used prosodic features such as **intonation** and stress appropriately. He spoke fluently and had normal **voice quality**. There was no evidence of phonological impairment. Sammy did not report any deterioration in his speech as a result of his recent illness and hospitalisation. His mother and sister also thought that his speech had remained unaltered following his illness.

Sammy obtained a phonemic or **letter fluency** score of 11 words in 60 seconds. This is slightly lower than might be expected based on published data. Gross et al. (2010) examined letter fluency in 588 men and women who participated in the Johns Hopkins Precursors Study – an investigation that examined associations between prospectively collected information about alcohol consumption ascertained on multiple occasions starting at age 55 years on average with domain-specific cognition at age 72 years.[13] The participants in this study were all graduates of the Johns Hopkins Medical School. The average letter fluency score for the letters F, A, S was 42.5 words (or 14.2 words for a single letter). ARBD is known to disrupt **executive function** skills.[14] It is likely that Sammy's score reflects some impairment of these cognitive skills and is consistent with his reduced performance on the MoCA.

Sammy displayed intact production and comprehension of **morphology**. He used inflectional and derivational morphemes with ease: *cruise liners* (plural inflectional suffix); *soft furnishings* (derivational suffix + plural inflectional suffix); *cheaper* (comparative inflectional suffix); and *concentration* (derivational suffix). Expressive and receptive **syntax** was also an area of strength in Sammy's communicative profile. Sammy was able to understand questions with complex syntax that were posed to him. In the following exchange, the author (INV) uses a question that contains subject–auxiliary inversion (underlined) and two **subordinate clauses**, one a **relative clause** (SC_1) and the other an **infinitive clause** (SC_2):

INV: <u>Do you have</u> any interests or hobbies [$_{SC_1}$that you like [$_{SC_2}$to pursue in your free time]]?
SAM: I'm just not fit enough [$_{SC_1}$to do [$_{SC_2}$what I want to do at the moment]]

Sammy's response reveals not only that he has understood what the author has asked him but also that he can make use of complex syntax. The utterance he uses in reply to the author also contains an infinitive clause (SC_1) and an interrogative subordinate clause (SC_2).

Sammy's lexical-semantic skills were relatively strong. When he omitted items or made errors during **confrontation naming**, his difficulties suggested a lack of prior exposure to target words and a possible effect of education on his naming. He was unable to attempt any response, for example, when shown pictures of uncommon vegetables like artichoke and asparagus. Other responses showed that he could provide a related, high-frequency lexical item in place of a low-frequency target word. When asked to name *French horn*, he responded "some sort of trumpet". When asked to be more specific, he replied "a bugle, some sort of wind instrument". Most of Sammy's naming errors, however, were visual in nature. For the picture of a pumpkin, he said "looks like a Terry's chocolate orange", only producing *pumpkin* when he was told that the target word occurred in the Cinderella story. Other visual errors included the following responses for the target words shown on the left of the arrows. In each case, there is a physical similarity, be it shape or markings, between the uttered word and the target word:

'skunk' → *badger*
'cherry' → *apple*
'chisel' → *paintbrush*
'lobster' → *locust* and *caterpillar*

Other naming errors were more clearly semantic in nature, such as the following examples:

'celery' → cauliflower (semantic field: vegetables)
'ant' → fly (semantic field: insects)
'rooster' → turkey (semantic field: bird)
'tiger' → leopard (semantic field: wild cat)
'lobster' → crab (semantic field: crustacean)

A range of cues successfully elicited target words that Sammy was struggling to produce. A gestural cue prompted his production of 'flute', while an orthographic cue (the letter R) elicited the production of 'racoon'. The picture of a tiger was eventually correctly named after use of an orthographic and a **phonemic cue. Semantic cues** were also used but were not always successful in eliciting production of a target word. For the target word 'pepper', the author used the following series of semantic cues. The first semantic cue produced no response. The second semantic cue produced a response that was not consistent with the first cue – pepperoni is a type of meat when Sammy was told the target word is a type of vegetable. It took a third semantic cue before the target word 'pepper' was produced:

Target word: *pepper*

'it's a type of vegetable' – no response
'it's on top of pizza' – responded 'pepperoni'
'it can be red, green or yellow' – responded 'pepper'

Sammy did not report any word-finding difficulties during conversation. However, his expressive language contained many indefinite **pronouns** like *somebody, anything* and *something* and other non-specific words like *stuff* and *thing*. Sammy used on average four of these words for every minute of his spoken contribution to the 42-minute audio-recording. The author used these same expressions a total of 16 times during the interaction, a rate which was less than half that displayed by Sammy. This may simply reflect Sammy's pre-morbid communication style, or it may suggest that he is having some **word-finding difficulty** after all. Several examples of Sammy's use of these expressions are shown below:

> I was doing also done cars car trimming and <u>stuff</u>
>
> *(conversation)*

> she's wringing out a cloth or <u>something</u>
>
> *(picture description)*

> "you know just concentration and <u>stuff</u> (.) is the <u>thing</u>
>
> *(conversation)*

That Sammy may have some difficulty with lexical access and retrieval is suggested by his performance on the semantic or **category fluency** task. Sammy produced 15 animal names in 60 seconds. Like **phonemic fluency**, this score is lower than might be expected based on published data. In the 588 participants in the Johns Hopkins Precursors Study, an average **semantic fluency** score of 18.3 animal names in 1 minute was obtained.[13] Horvat et al. (2015) recorded an average semantic fluency score of 22.3 animal names in 1 minute in 6,608 men and 22.2 animal names in 7,967 women, who were selected at random from population registers and electoral lists, and participated in the Health, Alcohol, and Psychosocial Factors in Eastern Europe prospective cohort study.[15] Sammy's superior semantic vs. phonemic fluency performance suggests that his difficulties with **letter fluency** cannot be accounted for by lexical access and retrieval problems alone – executive function deficits are making an independent contribution to these difficulties.

Aside from **lexical semantics**, Sammy was able to produce and understand meaningful sentences. His utterances contained different participant roles (e.g. **agent**, patient, **instrument**). Sammy was able to establish meaningful relations between phrases and **clauses** in sentences using **prepositions** and conjunctions that expressed a range of concepts. These concepts included *time* and *space* and complex relations such as those represented in italics below:

Reason: 'because'

> golfing trips were in Ireland '**cause** it was an Irish golfing society that I was playing with

Comparative: 'as'
> there's not the same quality **as** there used to be

Concessive: 'even though'

> **even though** ... probably where the drinkin' was concerned and stuff ah (1:65) you know you could have managed but you still weren't doing it right

Sammy displayed strengths and weaknesses in **pragmatics**. An area of pragmatic strength was his use and appreciation of **humour**. During the **confrontation naming** test, he responded with *crab* when shown the picture of a lobster, insisting they were 'the same thing'. He then went on to engage in humour based on the dual meaning of the word 'crab': a crustacean versus a slang term for a sexually transmitted infection:

> it's a lobster, a crab, it's the same thing, they are, but then if you've got the crabs, you don't say you've got the lobsters!

Sammy made context-appropriate use of laughter during banter with the author. Below, talk about slowing down with advancing age is punctuated with episodes of laughter:

SAM: you name it I just loved playing sports all the time
INV: right okay but you will get back into a lot of these things once you get recovered
SAM: might be a bit slower like but *(laughter)*
INV: well none of us are 20 any more, sure we're not? *(laughter)*
SAM: we think we are but, don't we? *(laughter)*

Sammy was able to identify and correct misunderstandings when they occurred. During conversation about his favourite movies, Sammy said he liked thrillers. The author incorrectly took this to include horror movies, a misunderstanding that was quickly corrected:

INV: what sort of movies or films do you like?
SAM: maybe action movies yeah things like that thriller, thriller movies and stuff like that
INV: right so thrillers and horrors
SAM: don't like horrors

In the following extract, the author clearly understood that Sammy went to Canada *for the purpose* of playing golf. However, this was also a misunderstanding that Sammy was able to identify and correct:

INV: that must have been some trip going off to Canada to play golf
SAM: I suppose it, it wasn't to play golf ... I ended up playing golf when I was there

To correct these misunderstandings, Sammy was able to monitor his hearer's mental states and identify when these states did not adequately represent the message that he wanted to convey. This suggests that at least some of Sammy's pragmatic language skills were supported by strong **theory of mind** (ToM) skills. This is further indicated by Sammy's revision of his utterance in the following extract. Sammy is aware that he has used the **pronoun** *they* without first establishing for the hearer a **referent** of this expression. Accordingly, he moves to repair his utterance by replacing the pronoun with the noun *people*:

INV: you're not bothered about anything to do with words
SAM: nawh <u>they</u> either get me, <u>people</u> either get me or they don't

In this example, Sammy displayed sensitivity to his hearer's ignorance of the referent of a pronoun in conversation. There were many other occasions in conversation where Sammy used pronouns in the knowledge that his hearer would be able to establish their referents in the prior **discourse** context. In the following exchange, the **demonstrative pronoun** *that* has as its referent the different jobs that Sammy undertook as an upholsterer. Moreover, the hearer may be expected to establish this list of jobs as the referent of the demonstrative pronoun:

INV: what sort of furniture did you upholster?
SAM: anything from (.) dining room chairs, settees (.) ah (1:83) just ordinary chairs, Parker Knolls everything, bar work, cruise liners (.) everything basically you can upholster, I was doing also done cars car trimming and stuff, all sorts of stuff like <u>that</u>

Sammy was also able to use a range of linguistic devices to achieve **cohesion** between utterances. Grammatical **ellipsis** was evident on several occasions during conversation, as the italicised extract in the following exchange illustrates:

INV: it'll all come together, won't it?
SAM: yeah, I'm sure it will [*all come together*] but it's just to keep my patience

Lexical substitution was another form of cohesion that was employed effectively by Sammy. In the extract below, he used *one* as a substitute for *horror* during conversation about movies that he enjoyed watching:

INV: you don't like horrors
SAM: I thought they would watch <u>one</u> it is was (*unintelligible*) but I wouldn't go out of my way to watch <u>one</u>

Pronominal reference too was used to achieve cohesion during Sammy's conversation with the author. Below, Sammy uses the pronoun *it* to refer to his upholstery business:

SAM: I had an <u>upholstery business</u> where I (1:08) refurbished furniture and built furniture
INV: and can you tell me a bit more about that? Did you enjoy it?
SAM: oh yeah, I liked <u>it</u>

Although Sammy displayed several intact pragmatic language skills, his cognitive problems related to his ARBD did cause high-level **discourse** difficulties. Sammy's retention of verbal information in **memory** was a significant problem. His immediate recall of the Sam and Fred story was particularly poor, even after it was read aloud to him twice. At the end of the test session, the story was read to him a third time. On this occasion, he was able to recall a few details:

Sam and Fred:

> well Sam and his brother (0:87) ah had a farm and ah (1:90) the storm broke out (1:62) and they needed help so (1:71) the local people arrived to give them help to get the animals in the shelter from the (.) whatever (2:28) and (1:74) that's it

During the Cookie Theft picture description task, Sammy was able to describe the main actions in the scene. However, his description was superficial in nature, omitting all mention of the characters' mental states. The children's behaviour was not described as stealing or deception. It is doubtful that Sammy even grasped the children's deceptive intentions. He overlooked, for example, the young girl's **gesture** to her brother, warning him to be quiet so that they could avoid detection by their mother. Sammy reported that the sink was 'leaking' but did not account for this in terms of the mother's distracted mental state – she was clearly daydreaming and had forgotten to turn off the tap. The omission of these key mental states suggested that Sammy had a rather limited appreciation of the content of the picture, reflected in his exclusive use of action-based language:

Cookie Theft:

> well Sammy's got their hand in the cookie jar for a start (0:76) as they're fallin' off the stool (.) and the other wee girl's trying to grab a cookie (0:99) the other woman's sink's leaking (1:37) she's wringing out a cloth or something it looks like (.) I dunno what's happening outside just looks like a garden (1:90) there's a cup (1:42) there's curtains that's, that's it basically[1]

That Sammy may have had difficulty with mental state **inferences** is suggested by his performance on the Cookie Theft task. That he may also have had difficulty with temporal-causal inferences is suggested by his performance on the Flowerpot Incident. Sammy asked the author twice if the pictures in this task were related to each other. It was clear from his account that he could not establish inferences between events in the six pictures. For example, he failed to appreciate that the object on the ground was the smashed flowerpot that had fallen from the balcony in an earlier picture. He misunderstood the scene where the man walked through a doorway with his dog. This was not to take the dog for a walk, but to enter the building so that he could remonstrate with the owner of the apartment. This misinterpretation suggested that he could not see a causal relationship between the picture where the man was struck on the head and the picture where he entered the building – the man entered the building *because* he wanted to lodge a complaint about the injury he sustained in the street.

Flowerpot Incident:

SAM: out for a walk with the dog with a walking stick plant falls on his head (1:04) knocks off the hat (2:73) second picture is it meant to be related?
INV: um hum
SAM: obviously they put their hat back on (1:77) ah dog's barkin' (2:09) ah that's about it (1:53) and the other one is don't know what that is (.) where what it's meant to be (0:75) on the ground the third picture is taking the dog through the door (.) for a walk (.) or back into the house (0:91) I don't know (0:81) fourth one is (1:38) hittin' at the door with a stick (1:01) dog beside him he's just come up the stairs (1:09) woman's come out to meet the dog with a bone (2:10) now (.) he kisses her hand in the sixth picture (1:17) and the dog runs away with the bone

As well as omission of temporal-causal inferences, Sammy also failed to draw inferences about the mental states of the characters in this cartoon sequence. No mention is made of the gentleman's anger or that he intends to remonstrate with the owner of the apartment. Sammy did not state that the woman gives the man's dog a bone because she wants to make amends for the injury he has sustained. In the absence of these mental state inferences, the actions of the characters appear to lack motivation and purpose.

Sammy was visited again by the author on 2 February 2020, nearly six months after the first visit. By this stage, the result of his liver ultrasound conducted on 16 August 2019 was known. The scan was unremarkable with no focal liver lesion or evidence of **cirrhosis**. However, Sammy's ongoing consumption of alcohol since the first visit had had further repercussions for his health. On 13 November 2019 he was admitted to Accident and Emergency. He had a **tonic–clonic seizure** at home that was witnessed by his brother. Sammy reported to medical staff that he had reduced his intake of alcohol before stopping suddenly. He was kept in hospital for observation. Sammy received intravenous Pabrinex and was started on a reducing course of Librium. He was confabulating during his stay in hospital and had peripheral neuropathy in his right foot. There was no further seizure activity during admission. He was discharged on 15 November 2019 and offered a review by the Alcohol Liaison Nurse which he declined as he was already under the supervision of a substance misuse team. Sammy's MoCA scores fluctuated with his drinking. He achieved a score of 26/30 on 20 September 2019, but following discharge from hospital he obtained a score of 21/30 (**mild cognitive impairment**) on 18 November 2019.

Given Sammy's ongoing difficulties with abstinence, it was decided that a 4-week residence in an Addiction Treatment Unit was warranted. Sammy was admitted to hospital on 5 December 2019 for detox prior to his placement in the unit. He reported to medical staff that he had been drinking daily – mostly Guinness but also shorts such as whisky – since his discharge from hospital on 15 November 2019. He had 4–5 Guinness the day before admission and was unable to recall his last alcohol-free day. Sammy was again treated with intravenous Pabrinex and a reducing dose of Librium. He was discharged on 9 December 2019 for immediate onward transfer to the Addiction Treatment Unit.

Sammy attended the Addiction Treatment Unit between 9 December 2019 and 20 January 2020. He left the unit and returned home for Christmas. He was re-admitted on 6 January 2020 to complete his course. On admission to the unit on 9 December 2019, his MoCA score was 25/30 (mild cognitive impairment). On 13 December 2019, it was 24/30 (mild cognitive impairment). The Addenbrooke's Cognitive Examination (ACE-III) was conducted on 15 December 2019. Sammy scored 85/100 (mild cognitive impairment), with most deficits in the **attention**, **memory** and visuospatial domains. On Sammy's return to the ward on 6 January 2020, his MoCA score was 29/30. A ward drug screen conducted on his return revealed that he had used cocaine and a benzodiazepine, diazepam 5 mg, over the Christmas break. He admitted to the use of both drugs. He risked early discharge from the unit by concealing a mobile phone on the ward. This was only avoided because he handed the phone over voluntarily to staff and there was no adverse impact of his behaviour on other inpatients or on group dynamics as the unit was relatively empty immediately after Christmas. He did not consume alcohol over Christmas. He attributed this to his use of disulfiram 200 mg (Antabuse), a drug used in the treatment of alcohol dependence. By the time Sammy was discharged from the unit on 20 January 2020, his MoCA score was 29/30.

Sammy had not consumed any alcohol for a period of 60 days (8 weeks 4 days) by the time of the author's second visit. Reflecting his improved cognitive status on the MoCA, Sammy performed well on the phonemic (letter) fluency task. His score of 18 words in 60 seconds placed him above normative scores for healthy individuals of similar age, gender and education.[16] This was a significant improvement on his earlier score of 11 words in 60 seconds and suggested some recovery of his **executive function** skills. However, his semantic (category) fluency score was largely unchanged at 14 words in 60 seconds (15 words on the author's first visit). This score is below normative scores for healthy individuals of similar age, gender and education as Sammy,[16] and suggest that the **lexical retrieval** and generative capacity tested in this task had not so easily rebounded.

Sammy produced 17 errors during confrontation naming, a slight increase from the 13 errors he committed during the author's first visit. Eight of his 17 naming errors were also errors in the first visit. As before, most of Sammy's naming errors were semantically related to the target word. Sammy used the **superordinate term** "some sort of insect" for the target word *ant*, before producing *fly*, a word in the same **semantic field** as the target. Words in the same semantic field were produced for several other target words:

'beetle' → *locust (semantic field: insect)*

'violin' → *bass (semantic field: musical instrument)*

'cherry' → *plum; peach (semantic field: fruit)*

'coat' → *cloak (semantic field: garments)*

'French horn' → *saxophone; trombone; trumpet (semantic field: musical instrument)*

'skunk' → *badger (semantic field: mammal)*

'chest of drawers' → *dressing table (semantic field: furniture)*

'duck' → *swan (semantic field: bird)*

'peach' → *apple (semantic field: fruit)*

'rooster' → *turkey (semantic field: bird)*

Sammy eventually named *skunk, chest of drawers, duck, peach* and *rooster* correctly without the use of cuing by the author. Semantic and **phonemic cues** elicited production of other target words such as *celery* (phonemic cue), *grasshopper* (phonemic cue) and *pepper* (semantic cue). The **semantic cue** "it's dark and red and you find it in cocktails" did not elicit the production of *cherry*, however. The target word *artichoke* was incorrectly named as "pineapple". This was likely to be a visual error rather than a word from the wrong semantic field. Sammy responded with "don't know" for both *asparagus* and *potato*, eventually naming *potato* correctly when he looked more closely at the picture. Sammy was also previously unable to name *asparagus* as it did not appear to be a vegetable he knew.

Sammy's immediate and delayed recall of verbal material was still an area of considerable difficulty, suggesting significant **memory** problems remained. After a first reading of the Sam and Fred story, Sammy produced the following narrative:

Sam and Fred: immediate recall after first reading

> Sam and Fred were brothers who farmed their own land right they had bad weather they had to bring in, it's basically not a good story to remember

On this first reading, Sammy recalled only the names of the brothers, the fact that they farmed their own land and that the weather was bad. After a second reading of the story, he recalled two further pieces of information, that the farmers had to get the animals in, and that other people helped them:

Sam and Fred: immediate recall after second reading

> Sam and Fred were brothers then they had the bad weather then they had to get the animals in then they had to get people to give them a hand to get the animals in they asked for help and basically that's about it

On delayed recall, Sammy did not use the brothers' names. However, he mentioned for the first time that there was a "big storm":

Sam and Fred: delayed recall

> The two farmers went to work at their land then there was a big storm and then they went and got some people to ask them to give them a hand to get their animals in and that's basically it

Sammy's memory problems were also having a significant impact on his daily life. He could no longer recall appointments, even regular appointments. He used a diary to aid his memory but often forgot to enter appointments in it. Sammy is taking daily medication. Remembering to take his three daily doses has been challenging for him, even though they are prepared as a pill roll, i.e. pre-prepared sachets of pills for different times of the day. He has put keys and documents in special places for safekeeping but then cannot remember where he put them. In conversation, Sammy does not have any difficulty recalling people's names or names of objects and places. However, if he has just been told something or if a plan of action is agreed, he will almost instantly forget it without several repetitions.

Sammy's recall was much stronger when information was also presented to him visually. He watched a short animation of the Little Red Riding Hood story. His narrative was complete and well-structured, quite unlike his narrative for the much shorter Sam and Fred story which is presented auditorily only. Sammy's superior recall of this story was no doubt also facilitated by the fact that it is a reasonably familiar fictional narrative. He even states this during his narration (see question (3) at chapter end). But not all visual information in pictures was readily understood by Sammy. He was once again unable to identify the broken flowerpot on the pavement during the Flowerpot Incident task. This suggested that Sammy was unable to draw a necessary **inference**, namely, that the falling flowerpot in one picture became the broken flowerpot in a later picture when it shattered on the ground. Sammy's failure to identify the broken flowerpot, at least initially, suggests that he was still having difficulty establishing temporal-causal relations between depicted events in a narrative.

Flowerpot Incident:

> I dunno what that is on the ground haven't got a clue somebody's drawing's not very good
> I don't know what that is on the ground, oh it's the broken plant pot

Other **discourse** problems related to Sammy's cognitive difficulties concerned the attribution of mental states to characters in a story or scene. Sammy incorrectly characterised the mental state of the mother in the Cookie Theft picture description task. The sink was not overflowing because the mother was distracted by the children's behaviour. In fact, she was completely unaware of their behaviour *and* the overflowing sink *because* she was daydreaming:

Cookie Theft:

> the mother reacts probably as she's overflowing the tap in the kitchen with the distraction that's goin' on

In the Flowerpot Incident, Sammy was also unable to make sense of the complex mental states that motivated the gentleman to kiss the elderly woman on the hand. First, he explicitly states that he does not know why the gentleman would perform such an action when the woman has just dropped a plant pot on him. Clearly, he kisses her hand as a means of expressing his gratitude to her for the kindness she has shown in giving his dog a bone:

> I don't know, she's only after dropping the plant pot and then he's kissing her on the hand

Then, he attributes an incorrect intention to the gentleman, namely, that he is seeking to go out for a night with the woman:

> then he kisses on her hand and probably asks her to go out for a night out with him for a bit of craic

That mental state inferences were still a problem for Sammy on this second visit indicates that any improvement in cognitive skills since the author's first visit has not extended to the domain of **social cognition**.

COMMUNICATION PROFILE:

Speech intelligibility:

- Sammy did not have a motor speech disorder and his speech was fully intelligible; all aspects of speech production and phonology were intact.

Morphology and syntax:

- Sammy displayed intact morphology and used a range of inflectional and derivational morphemes; he was able to use and understand utterances with complex syntax.

Vocabulary and semantics:

- Lexical-semantic impairments were evident in expressive language; some errors during confrontation naming suggested an effect of education, other errors were visual and semantic in nature; cues facilitated naming; Sammy did not report word-finding difficulties in conversation but did make excessive use of indefinite pronouns and words like 'stuff' and 'thing'; reduced semantic fluency for animal names; Sammy expressed complex conceptual relations in sentences.

Pragmatics:

- Sammy was able to use and appreciate humour; laughter was used appropriately in conversation; could identify when misunderstandings occurred in conversation and moved to correct them; was sensitive to his hearer's knowledge and ignorance during conversation; had good topic management; used normal turn-taking and other skills of conversation management.

Discourse:

- Sammy showed good use of cohesive devices including ellipsis, lexical substitution and pronominal reference; had difficulty using mental state inferences and temporal-causal inferences during discourse production; his omission of information in discourse related to poor recall of verbal material.

Cognition:

- Sammy's performance on the MoCA indicated moderate cognitive impairment improving to mild impairment before discharge from hospital; reduced phonemic fluency (poorer than semantic fluency), suggesting executive function deficits; impaired immediate recall of verbal material; Sammy reported poor concentration and frustration at not being able to concentrate.

Suggestions for Further Reading

(1) Zahr, N.M., Kaufman, K.L. and Harper, C.G. (2011) 'Clinical and pathological features of alcohol-related brain damage', *Nature Reviews. Neurology*, 7:
284–294. doi: 10.1038/nrneurol.2011.42

In this review, the authors examine ARBD from the perspective of WE
and KS, two better characterised neurological concomitants of alcoholism.
The review addresses the clinical presentations, postmortem brain pathology, in vivo MRI findings, and molecular mechanisms associated with these
conditions.

(2) Thomson, A.D., Guerrini, I., Bell, D., Drummond, C., Duka, T., Field, M.,
Kopelman, M., Lingford-Hughes, A., Smith, I., Wilson, K. and Marshall, E.J.
(2012) 'Alcohol-related brain damage: Report from a Medical Council on
Alcohol Symposium, June 2010', *Alcohol and Alcoholism*, 47 (2): 84–91.

With short contributions from all eleven authors, this report examines
many aspects of ARBD, including the role of thiamine deficiency in WE,
cognitive dysfunction in alcoholics, and clinical, neuroimaging and neuropsychological findings in KS.

(3) Royal College of Psychiatrists. (2014) *Alcohol and Brain Damage in Adults:
With Reference to High-Risk Groups*. London: Author.

This 90-page report of the Royal College of Psychiatrists in the UK
addresses many aspects of ARBD and related syndromes. Readers are
referred to the sections on clinical definition and diagnosis of ARBD (pp.
14–21), epidemiology of ARBD (pp. 22–24) and the neurobiological basis
of WKS and ARBD (pp. 25–29). The full college report is available online at:
https://www.rcpsych.ac.uk/docs/default-source/improving-care/better-
mh-policy/college-reports/college-report-cr185.pdf?sfvrsn=66534d91_2

Questions

(1) Sammy claimed that he was familiar with the Cinderella story. However,
he was unable to tell any part of the story even after using the pictures in a
wordless picture book to jog his memory. The author then told the story to
him as they both viewed the pictures in the book. Sammy then went on to
give the following narrative. Examine this narrative in detail and answer the
questions below:

> well she's out (1:58) with a horse (.) and him (1:37) I feel so stupid so
> I do now, and ah (3:35) she wants to go to the ball she meets the old
> woman ends up the fairy godmother (1:09) sh, sh, she turns a pump-
> kin into a (0:93) a carriage (1:89) takes her to the ball and she has a
> lovely gets a lovely dress glass shoes (1:17) and she dances with the
> prince all night (1:45) then she has to be home before twelve (0:77)

so (0:88) in her haste to get home she drops a glass slipper (0:79) on the step (1:34) and she gets home (.) and she's only one slipper on her (1:60) then the prince wants to find out who she is so he sends his courtier out (1:07) look round the (0:84) as a province whatever it's called and finds her and tries it on her and fits perfectly (1:76) and ah (3:01) then he finds out who she is (1:61) end up (.) they get married and live happily ever after

(a) Sammy omits considerable information from his narrative. However, the omission is most marked in one part of his narrative. Which part is this?

(b) Sammy shifts the referent of the pronoun *she* at one point in the narrative without signalling this shift of reference. Where does this occur?

(c) The utterance "she drops a glass slipper on the step" is well-formed. However, it falls short of a hearer's expectation that an utterance should be maximally informative. In what way is this utterance not fully informative?

(d) Sammy uses lexical reiteration as a form of cohesion. Identify where this occurs in his narrative.

(e) What feature of this narrative suggests that Sammy has retained knowledge of the conventional structure of a fictional narrative?

(2) Sammy completed two procedural discourse tasks, namely, how to make a sandwich and how to write a letter to someone. His responses to each of these tasks are shown below:

Making a sandwich:

well you need your bread okay (0:67) you need your butter and cheese and ham you butter the bread depends whether the ham's sliced or not (.) say it is you put the ham on cut up cheese put it on put the (.) other bit of bread on top buttered (.) and if you like butter that is and (.) cut it in half and eat it

Writing a letter:

go and get the bit of paper (1:22) sit down and think about what we're going to write in the letter (0:60) and start off to beginning (0:79) just (1:78) hello (1:06) and (1:53) write a letter an either (.) I just feel (0:76) is this before you post the letter or do this post the letters [*INV: just keep going*] write the letter put it in an envelope (.) put a stamp on it and post it put a name on it

(a) Are there any sequencing errors in Sammy's discourse? If so, identify where they occur.

(b) What feature of Sammy's sandwich-making discourse suggests he is aware that his instructions are conditional in nature and may be subject to change?

(c) Does Sammy check his understanding of task instructions at any point? If so, what does this behaviour reveal about his cognitive and language skills?

(d) What type of cohesive device does Sammy use in the following extract from the sandwich-making discourse?

> depends whether the ham's sliced or not (.) say it is you put the ham on

(e) Sammy is clearly adept at describing routine activities like making a sandwich and writing a letter. His procedural discourse is significantly superior to his narrative discourse. Give *three* reasons that might explain why this is the case.

(3) During the author's second visit to Sammy, he watched a short animation of the story of Little Red Riding Hood. Sammy then retold the story. The narrative he produced is shown in full below. Examine it in detail and then answer the questions below:

> Well, Little Red Riding Hood she has her wee cape on her and her wee red hood, and her mother asked her to take her granny over some food of some description, I don't know what it was, so on her way over there she bumps into the wolf, and the wolf asks her where she was going and she says to her grandmother's, so off she skips and the wolf goes a shorter way to get to the grandmother's, knocks the door, puts on a lighter voice, grandmother invites the wolf in, and the wolf eats her up and puts her clothes on and gets into bed, by the time eh the grandmother by the time little miss Riding Hood got there, she knocked the door and the wolf let her in, and she comes into the room and she says "what a big nose you've got", "all the better to smell you with", I think, "what big ears you've got", "all the better to hear you with", I think that was I'm just relying on the nursery rhyme I don't know, "what big teeth you've", "all the better to eat you at", and then he jumped out of the bed and ate her up, and then he got back into bed and started sleeping, then the woodcutter who heard the cries came to the house with his axe, and killed the wolf and out popped the grandmother and Little Red Riding Hood, and so they were safe and then the woodcutter marches off with his axe and the skin of the wolf over his shoulder

(a) Sammy produced a cohesive narrative. Using examples, identify *two* types of cohesive device that he uses in his narrative.

(b) With *two* exceptions, Sammy makes appropriate lexical selections. Identify the two occasions where Sammy should have made a different lexical selection.

(c) Sammy uses direct and indirect reported speech. Identify *one* example of each type of reported speech in his narrative.

(d) Sammy engages in repair during this narrative. Identify where he undertakes repair. What type of repair strategy have you identified?

(e) Sammy engages in meta-discourse at two points in his narrative. Identify where this occurs. What does the use of meta-discourse reveal about Sammy's cognitive-linguistic skills?

Answers

(1) (a) Sammy omits the entire first half of the narrative. He picks up the story at the point where Cinderella meets the fairy godmother. However, when he gets the story underway at this point, he succeeds in including all main details until the end.

(b) When Sammy states "she turns a pumpkin into a (0:93) a carriage (1:89) takes her to the ball and she has a lovely gets a lovely dress glass shoes", the first use of the pronoun *she* refers to the fairy godmother while the second use refers to Cinderella. However, this shift of reference is not explicitly signalled by Sammy. A hearer who is unfamiliar with the story of Cinderella would assume that the second use of the pronoun *she* also refers to the fairy godmother.

(c) The utterance is not fully informative because Sammy does not state that Cinderella drops a glass slipper on the step *of the palace*. The omission of this information makes Sammy's well-formed utterance less informative than a hearer might expect to be the case.

(d) In lexical reiteration, a synonym or near-synonym of a word or phrase is used to link consecutive utterances. Sammy uses lexical reiteration when he varies *glass shoes* with *glass slippers* in the following extract: "she has a lovely gets a lovely dress glass shoes [...] in her haste to get home she drops a glass slipper (0:79) on the step".

(e) Sammy concludes his narrative by saying that Cinderella and the prince "live happily ever after". This is a conventional closing sequence to a fictional narrative.

(2) (a) During his letter-writing discourse, Sammy makes a sequencing error when he states that the addressee's name is put on the envelope *after* the letter has been posted.

(b) Sammy introduces two qualifications into his sandwich-making discourse: "depends whether the ham's sliced or not" and "if you like butter that is". These qualifications describe conditions that may alter the instructions that Sammy is setting out.

(c) During his letter-writing discourse, Sammy asks the author if the task relates only up to the point "before you post the letter". This suggests that he is able to monitor his verbal output and ensure that his instructions fulfil the examiner's expectations regarding relevance and informativeness.

(d) Sammy uses grammatical ellipsis in this utterance: "depends whether the ham's sliced or not (.) say it is [*sliced*]".

(e) (i) Making a sandwich and writing a letter are well-rehearsed activities. The procedural discourses that capture these activities are likely to activate well-established scripts. These scripts are less likely to be in place for fictional and other narratives; (ii) the procedural discourses for these activities each describe only four or five stages. Even short narratives usually contain more than four or five elements for speakers to recall and then organise into a coherent whole; (iii) procedural discourses that set out task instructions must capture causal and temporal relations between steps. Temporal-causal relations are only one set of relations that must be represented in narratives. Typically, narratives must also represent the intentional states of characters.

(3) (a) lexical reiteration (bold) and anaphoric reference (underlining): "<u>grandmother</u> invites the **wolf** in, and the **wolf** eats <u>her</u> up"

(b) Sammy uses *lighter* voice instead of *higher* voice. He also uses *nursery rhyme* instead of *fairy tale*.

(c) direct reported speech: "she comes into the room and she says "what a big nose you've got""; indirect reported speech: "the wolf asks her where she was going".

(d) repair: "by the time eh the grandmother by the time little miss Riding Hood got there"; this is self-initiated self-repair.

(e) Sammy engages in meta-discourse when he remarks of the food that Red Riding Hood carried to her grandmother "I don't know what it was". He uses further meta-discourse when he states: "I think that was, I'm just relying on the nursery rhyme, I don't know". The ability to engage in meta-discourse suggests that Sammy can temporarily suspend his discourse and provide commentary on some aspect of it (e.g. his lack of knowledge of the specific foods for the grandmother).

Note

1 It should be noted that the use of a plural possessive determiner (*their*) and plural personal pronoun (*they*) to describe one person is a grammatical feature of Sammy's dialect and is not a sign of grammatical disorder:

Sammy's got <u>their</u> hand (*Cookie theft*)
<u>they're</u> fallin' off (*Cookie theft*)
<u>they</u> put <u>their</u> hat back on (*Flowerpot incident*)

References

[1] Zahr, N.M., Kaufman, K.L. and Harper, C.G. (2011) 'Clinical and pathological features of alcohol-related brain damage', *Nature Reviews Neurology*, 7: 284–294. doi:10.1038/nrneurol.2011.42

[2] Thomson, A.D., Guerrini, I., Bell, D., Drummond, C., Duka, T., Field, M., Kopelman, M., Lingford-Hughes, A., Smith, I., Wilson, K. and Marshall, E.J. (2012) 'Alcohol-related brain damage: Report from a Medical Council on Alcohol Symposium, June 2020', *Alcohol and Alcoholism*, 47 (2): 84–91.

[3] Gilchrist, G. and Morrison, D.S. (2005) 'Prevalence of alcohol related brain damage among homeless hostel dwellers in Glasgow', *European Journal of Public Health*, 15 (6): 587–588.

[4] Smith, I.P. and Flanigan, C. (2000) 'Korsakoff's psychosis in Scotland: Evidence for increased prevalence and regional variation', *Alcohol and Alcoholism*, 35 (1): 8–10.

[5] Royal College of Psychiatrists (2014) *Alcohol and Brain Damage In Adults With Reference To High-Risk Groups.* London: Author.

[6] National Organization for Rare Disorders (2005) *Wernicke-Korsakoff syndrome.* https://rarediseases.org/rare-diseases/wernicke-korsakoff-syndrome/. Accessed 20 October 2019.

[7] Harper, C.G., Sheedy, D.L., Lara, A.I., Garrick, T.M., Hilton, J.M. and Raisanen, J. (1998) 'Prevalence of Wernicke-Korsakoff syndrome in Australia: Has thiamine fortification made a difference?', *Medical Journal of Australia*, 168 (11): 542–545.

[8] Sanvisens, A., Zuluaga, P., Fuster, D., Rivas, I., Tor, J., Marcos, M., Chamorro, A.J. and Muga, R. (2017) 'Long-term mortality of patients with an alcohol-related Wernicke-Korsakoff syndrome', *Alcohol and Alcoholism*, 52 (4): 466–471.

[9] Ridley, N.J., Draper, B. and Withall, A. (2013) 'Alcohol-related dementia: An update of the evidence', *Alzheimer's Research & Therapy*, 5: 3. http://alzres.com/content/5/1/3.

[10] Gerridzen, I.J., Moerman-van den Brink, W.G., Depla, M.F., Verschuur, E.M., Veenhuizen, R.B., van der Wouden, J.C., Hertogh, C.M. and Joling, K.J. (2017) 'Prevalence and severity of behavioural symptoms in patients with Korsakoff syndrome and other alcohol-related cognitive disorders: A systematic review', *International Journal of Geriatric Psychiatry*, 32 (3): 256–273.

[11] Harper, C.G., Giles, M. and Finlay-Jones, R. (1986) 'Clinical signs in the Wernicke-Korsakoff complex: A retrospective analysis of 131 cases diagnosed at necropsy', *Journal of Neurology, Neurosurgery, and Psychiatry*, 49 (4): 341–345.

[12] Montanez, A., Ruskin, J.N., Hebert, P.R., Lamas, G.A. and Hennekens, C.H. (2004) 'Prolonged QTc interval and risks of total and cardiovascular mortality and sudden death in the general population: A review and qualitative overview of the prospective cohort studies', *Archives of Internal Medicine*, 164 (9): 943–948.

[13] Gross, A.L., Rebok, G.W., Ford, D.E., Chu, A.Y., Gallo, J.J., Liang, K.-Y., Meoni, L.A., Shihab, H.M., Wang, N.-Y. and Klag, M.J. (2010) 'Alcohol consumption and domain-specific cognitive function in older adults: Longitudinal data from the Johns Hopkins Precursors Study', *Journal of Gerontology: Psychological Sciences*, 66B (1): 39–47.

[14] de la Monte, S.M. and Kril, J.J. (2014) 'Human alcohol-related neuropathology', *Acta Neuropathologica*, 127 (1): 71–90.

[15] Horvat, P., Richards, M., Kubinova, R., Pajak, A., Malyutina, S., Shishkin, S., Pikhart, H., Peasey, A., Marmot, M.G., Singh-Manoux, A. and Bobak, M. (2015) 'Alcohol consumption, drinking patterns, and cognitive function in older Eastern European adults', *Neurology*, 84 (3): 287–295.

[16] Tombaugh, T.N., Kozak, J. and Rees, L. (1999) 'Normative data stratified by age and education for two measures of verbal fluency: FAS and animal naming', *Archives of Clinical Neuropsychology*, 14 (2): 167–177.

CASE STUDY 9

Covid-19 Infection

KEY FACTS AND FIGURES:

- Covid-19 is a disease caused by a novel coronavirus that first came to prominence in December 2019, following an outbreak of severe respiratory illness in the central Chinese city of Wuhan. The virus has a zoonotic origin, most probably bats, with Malayan pangolins a likely intermediate host.[1] Along with the viruses that cause SARS (severe acute respiratory syndrome) and MERS (Middle East respiratory syndrome), novel coronavirus is the third beta coronavirus to infect humans.
- Human-to-human transmission occurs primarily by means of droplets and fomites (i.e. objects and materials that are likely to carry infection such as clothes and utensils). The faecal-oral route is not thought to be a major driver of transmission.
- Risk factors for severe Covid-19 disease include age (greater risk $\geq$ 65 years), sex (greater risk in males), ethnicity (greater risk in people from Black and minority ethnic communities) and the presence of underlying health conditions (e.g. diabetes, hypertension). In patients with severe Covid-19 disease requiring hospitalisation, the mortality rate is high. In one study, 32 of 52 (61.5%) critically ill patients had died at 28 days, with the median duration from admission to the intensive care unit to death seven days.[2]
- Symptoms of Covid-19 appear between two and 14 days after exposure to the virus. Originally thought to include fever, cough and shortness of breath, the symptoms of Covid-19 have been expanded to include

DOI: 10.4324/9781003153559-10

fatigue, muscle or body aches, headache, new loss of taste or smell (anosmia), sore throat, congestion or runny nose, nausea or vomiting, and diarrhoea. There is some evidence that people who are asymptomatic or presymptomatic can transmit the virus.[3,4]

- Neurological symptoms are common in people with Covid-19 infection. In one systematic review, headache, dizziness, taste and smell dysfunctions, and impaired consciousness were the most frequently reported neurological symptoms, found in 20.1%, 6.8%, 50.8%, 59.2% and 5.1%, respectively, of the populations studied.[5] Cognitive impairments in memory, attention and executive function are also reported.[6,7]

Background

Pauline (not her real name) is 48;8 years old. She is single and has no children. Pauline is a consultant clinical nurse specialist in urology in the UK. This role involves clinical and educational responsibilities, with some organisational work also. She has 17 years of formal education. In 1994, Pauline obtained a diploma in nursing. In 1997, she graduated with a BSc (Hons) in Professional Development in Nursing with District Nursing. She obtained a MSc in Health and Wellbeing with Urology/Continence in 2011. In 2019, Pauline qualified as a non-medical prescriber.

Pauline had high exposure to Covid-19 through her work as a nurse. In March and April 2020, she was supporting a care home of 31 residents, 19 of whom initially tested positive for Covid-19. On the island where Pauline lives and works, there were 13 deaths related to Covid-19. Pauline directly cared for 11 of these 13 patients. In the second week in April 2020, Pauline developed fatigue, a cough, sore eyes, bowel symptoms and a loss of taste. She had swab tests for Covid 19 on 14 April, 23 April and 5 June, all of which were negative. On 24 June, a positive antibody test result confirmed that she had been exposed to the virus. This test was repeated on 2 December 2020 and antibodies were still present. Pauline reports that at least two-thirds of the nurses she works with had either positive Covid-19 swabs or a positive antibody test.

Prior to contracting Covid-19, Pauline described her general state of health as good. She had a **tonsillectomy** in 1995 and an emergency **cholecystectomy** in 2017. She has **hypertension** for which she takes medication. Pauline reports that she is slightly overweight for her age, gender and height. She has no allergies to food or medication. Her hearing and vision are normal. She does not consume alcohol and does not smoke or vape. She describes her diet as good although thinks she could probably eat fewer sweets. She takes daily multivitamins and a hair and nail supplement. Pauline takes regular exercise. She swims six days a week and enjoys cycling. She does not believe that she has a healthy work–life balance. Pauline reports working too much and experiences fatigue from work.

She enjoys swimming, boating and gardening, and looking after her three cats and five tortoises. She meets friends socially on a weekly basis and uses WhatsApp to communicate with people.

Clinical Symptoms

Pauline has experienced a wide array of symptoms related to Covid-19 infection. She has had severe fatigue and **conjunctivitis**. She reports severe pins and needles in her limbs, a sensation that she describes as "fizzing". Pauline has also developed significant **memory** loss. She cannot remember the names of people and objects and often forgets appointments and plans that she has made. She must write everything down. At work, she forgets the times and dates of patient appointments, and must phone patients to confirm their appointments. She forgets meetings and mixes up the days of meetings. She can also forget to pay bills, and often believes she has already paid them when this is not the case. Pauline had no difficulty with her memory prior to Covid-19 infection. "I was always on the ball", she reports.

Among her moderate symptoms are gastrointestinal problems (viz., loose bowel motions) and a loss of taste and smell. She has experienced mild coughing, aches and pains, and headache. Pauline has not experienced several symptoms commonly identified with Covid-19 infection, including fever, breathing difficulties, sore throat, and chest pain or pressure. She has not had a skin rash or ear infections. Pauline did not take any medication for her symptoms.

Pauline was not under any medical supervision while she had Covid-19 and is not currently receiving any medical treatment or monitoring. On 11 August 2020, she had a chest X-ray which was normal. Pauline feels that her occupational exposure to Covid-19 has had an adverse effect on her mental health. She has received psychological support following her experience of nursing so many people who died of the infection in the care home where she worked. Pauline thinks her recovery from Covid-19 has been slow, probably because she was working instead of resting when she had the virus. Although her fatigue and memory loss are still very severe, she reports some improvement in the "fizzing" sensation in her limbs. Given the persistence of her symptoms over many months since her acute Covid illness, Pauline fits the definition of "**long Covid**".

Daily Activities

Pauline reports a significant impact of Covid-19 infection on her daily life. Prior to becoming infected, Pauline described her job as "very busy and consuming but very rewarding". There were never enough hours in the day to fit everything in, she reports. Since becoming unwell, she has had to reduce her hours of work as she is too fatigued to work full time. Pauline is contracted to work a 37.5-hour week, although she usually works about 40 hours. Following Covid-19 infection, she has had to reduce her working week to 60% of her normal hours. Currently, she is trying to increase her hours back up to 37.5 hours per week. She worked 22 hours per week for the first three weeks. This increased to 29 hours per week for the next three weeks.

Prior to becoming unwell, Pauline undertook intensive, daily exercise. Her level of physical activity has been compromised by her illness. Every Monday and Wednesday, she used to swim for 40–60 minutes in the morning and then cycle three miles to and from work. Now she can either swim or cycle, but not do both. Every Tuesday and Thursday, she would cycle the three miles to and from work. She still tries to do this. Every Friday, Pauline would swim in the pool in the morning for 45–60 minutes, swim for 20 minutes in the sea, and in the evening do 1 hour of pool training. She can now only do one swim on a Friday, and this tends to be the sea swim. Starting 28 September 2020, Pauline has managed to undertake her normal exercise routine. However, she describes herself as "shattered" in the evenings.

Pauline has also had to reduce social and leisure activities. She cannot undertake anything that requires a late night. If she is going for a meal, this needs to be done early in the evening. She has lost the motivation to undertake household chores and reports needing to pace herself.

Medication

Pauline is on several prescribed medications. She takes perindopril 4 mg once a day for the treatment of **hypertension**. Pauline uses the hormone replacement therapies Utrogestan 200 mg (days 15–26 of cycle) and Oestrogel, a gel the size of a 50-pence piece nightly. Once a day, she takes Calcichew (a calcium supplement) and ferrous sulphate 200 mg (an iron supplement). Because of her high-risk occupation, Pauline was among the first people in the UK to receive the Covid-19 vaccine. She received her first shot on 21 December 2020 and her second shot on 11 January 2021.

Communication

Pauline's self-reported cognitive problems since contracting Covid-19 have had a negative impact on communication. When she is talking to others, she frequently struggles to remember the names of people and things. Pauline's concentration is limited. She must really focus during conversation in order to follow what others are saying. She frequently loses concentration and her train of thought. Her fatigue has made it difficult for her to follow the plot in a story or a film. Pauline reports forgetting how to spell words. At times, she has no energy or motivation to engage with people. Although she communicates every day with people at work and outside work, she now must make an effort to communicate with people outside work.

The author spoke to Pauline online on 19 October 2020. It was 11 a.m. UK time. The conversation lasted an hour. Pauline was sitting comfortably in her living room, with her computer resting on the arm of the sofa. There was adequate daylight in the room for viewing pictures on the screen, and Pauline wore her glasses throughout the session. She was alert and responsive and coped well with interruptions caused by the technology and the delivery of mail by a postman. Pauline had a relaxed demeanour and appeared happy to talk about her work and her recent Covid illness. She did not display frustration during the completion of tasks even when she encountered more struggle than she might have expected.

Pauline's speech was fully intelligible. Her production of speech sounds was accurate, and she had normal speech **resonance** and **voice quality**. Pauline displayed adequate respiratory support for speech and good vocal volume, and her **intonation** and stress were in the normal range. Pauline's speech was fluent, and her speaking rate was normal. She did not have **dysarthria** or **apraxia of speech**, and there was no evidence of a phonological impairment.

Given that SARS-CoV-2 is a new pathogen, there is little published research on the implications of Covid-19 for language and cognition. The debilitating fatigue that Pauline and other people with **long Covid** have experienced finds parallels with **chronic fatigue syndrome**, a condition in which language and cognitive problems have been documented.[8,9,10] Pauline's self-reported cognitive-linguistic difficulties are supported by her performance in several language tasks. Her use and understanding of **morphology** and **syntax** appeared intact for the most part. Pauline was able to use a range of morphological structures in her expressive language, including prefixes and inflectional and **derivational suffixes**:

what was going to happen and where we'd be <u>re</u>deployed

(prefix)

they weren't <u>un</u>comfort<u>able</u>

(prefix + derivational suffix)

we had end-of-life medic<u>ations</u>

(derivational suffix + inflectional suffix)

what we found the hard<u>est</u> thing

(inflectional suffix)

Pauline also made use of complex syntax in spontaneous conversation such as **passive voice** constructions and embedded **clauses**:

we decided <u>that we would work three nights a week</u>

(that-clause)

people <u>that were younger, healthier bodied and healthy hearts</u>, it might have been different

(*relative clause*)

one of the care homes <u>had been closed</u> because 80% of their staff had come back positive

(*passive voice construction*)

<u>what we found the hardest thing</u> was when em (.) the virus it took people so quickly

(*nominal relative clause*)

Syntactic difficulties emerged when Pauline was presented with words and was asked to form brief sentences. Her overall accuracy during sentence generation was 50%. Errors occurred at the three- and four-word level. Pauline struggled with the combined demands of holding words in **working memory** whilst assembling them into a well-formed sentence. For the four words <*forest, mushroom, pick, wild*>, Pauline produced the following utterance:

If you go into the forest and pick some wild mushrooms

Pauline's comprehension of syntax was intact for conversation. She understood the syntax of the following utterances used by the author:

it's incredible <u>you ended up with three false negative tests</u>

(*subordinate clause*)

I've heard people say that it feels as if [your brain <u>is being stabbed</u> by that thing]

(*passive voice construction in an embedded clause*)

In terms of **semantics**, Pauline occasionally used an **argument structure** that misrepresented participants and events in **discourse**. During the Sam and Fred story, she stated that *the door opened*. No external force is seen to act on the *door* which has the **semantic role** of patient in the sentence. In the actual story, however, it was the storm that ripped open the door of the barn. Because Pauline does not assign *storm* to the semantic role of natural force, her representation of this event lacks causation:

The door [PATIENT] opened.

The storm [NATURAL FORCE] ripped open the door [PATIENT] of the barn.

Naming was an area of strength for Pauline. She achieved 90% accuracy during **confrontation naming**. The only pictures that she could not name were *racoon* and *French horn*, both of which could be explained by a lack of familiarity with the animal and musical instrument, respectively. Her **category fluency** scores of 25 animal names and 17 names of fruit in 60 seconds place her above normative scores (means) for people of similar age, education level and gender.[11,12] Her confrontation naming and category fluency performances suggest strong lexical access, retrieval and generation. And yet Pauline reported **word-finding difficulty** in conversation. Although there was not clear evidence of word-finding difficulties in Pauline's expressive language (but see *Sam and Fred* below), she did make extensive use of the **filler** *em* at syntactic boundaries and before **noun phrases**. It is possible that some general slowing of information processing was at the source of Pauline's word-finding difficulty, and that her use of this filler secured her additional time in which to retrieve words and plan her utterances:

Conversation:

> my job involves **em** clinical work so that's seein' patients with urology continence problems **em** I'm also involved in teach, teachin' so I teach pre-reg and post-reg **em** nursing students **em** I'm involved in organisational issues **em** within the within our health service **em** I do ah I participate nationally and speak at national conferences **em** I write journal articles

That cognitive limitations affected Pauline's use of language was evident in her immediate and delayed recall of the 100-word Sam and Fred story. On immediate recall, Pauline produced only 50% of the information that was necessary to convey the full content of the story. This figure dropped to 25% on delayed recall. As the extract below illustrates, Pauline omitted temporal references – *thirty years* and *by midnight* – in her immediate recall of the story. She also omitted key events (e.g. *the crops were washed away*) and produced several incomplete propositions (e.g. *the door [of what?] opened*). Pauline occasionally used general **lexemes** (*people* and *animals*) in place of more specific words (*villagers* and *cows and sheep*). Her use of 'came out' lacks the specificity of the verb *escaped*. These features combined resulted in a narrative that was under-informative and vague with respect to the original version:

Immediate recall:

> there was the two brothers Sam and Fred em they'd had their farm for many years you did tell me but I can't remember em they had a storm one night and em during the storm the door opened (1.21) and lots of their

animals ah I think it was sheep that they had came out and em the village the village nearby or the people came to help them and em helped them with the animals put them back

When Pauline was able to activate the script of a well-known fictional narrative, namely, the Cinderella story, the informativeness of her story telling increased to 64%. That said, **memory** problems alone cannot account for Pauline's omission of information during **discourse** production. During the Cookie Theft picture description task, the picture remains on view and details do not need to be committed to memory. Once again, however, Pauline related only 50% of the content in the picture. Pauline succeeded in describing fully the actions of the boy in the scene. But there is no mention of what the mother is doing beyond a description of her as being distracted and the young girl's actions are omitted altogether. Pauline's description suggests that other cognitive deficits, possibly affecting **attention** and concentration, may have a role to play in her language difficulties. Pauline reports that her ability to concentrate has been limited since she contracted Covid-19:

Cookie theft:

so there's em there's a lady looks like the mother (4.30) distracted by something outside in and the wash hand the sink is overflowing em there's two children little boy and girl little boy's on a stool and he's trying to steal some cookies out of the cookie jar and he's nearly going to fall off the stool em you can see (*unintelligible*) out the window (3.54) and looks like another little house

Deficits in attention and concentration may also account for Pauline's misidentification of the falling flowerpot as a bucket of water in the Flowerpot Incident narrative. This is another discourse production task in which Pauline was underinformative, relating only 30% of the information that is essential to the story. The stimulus pictures remain in front of the examinee, again eliminating the need to commit the content of the pictures to memory. Pauline's consistent lack of informativeness and misidentification of objects in the absence of demands on memory suggest that there may be some compromise of her **executive function** skills, leading to a reduction in the efficiency with which she attends to, and gleans information from, pictured stimuli. That Pauline has some **executive dysfunction** is suggested by her **letter fluency** score. She was only able to produce a total of 29 words beginning with the letters F, A and S. This is well below mean scores for people of similar age, education level and gender to Pauline:[11]

Age (40–49 years): 43.5 words
Education (17–21 years): 43.9 words
Gender (female): 37.8 words

The post-Covid fatigue reported by Pauline and other people with **long Covid** has similarities to **chronic fatigue syndrome**, a condition in which letter fluency, attention and concentration are also known to be impaired.[13,14,15]

Notwithstanding her executive function difficulties in attention and concentration, Pauline was able to plan and organise **discourse**. She correctly sequenced all events in the Cinderella story, a complex narrative that requires the integration of many individual stages. When asked to describe the steps involved in writing a letter to someone, Pauline began by talking about the layout of the letter itself. However, she realised she had forgotten the first stage – getting notepaper and a pen – and promptly repaired her utterance at the point marked ↑:

> on the right side well I ạ notepaper and pen and I would, I would get one
> ↑
> with lines on it

Pauline displayed strengths in another cognitive area, namely, **theory of mind**. She attributed cognitive and **affective mental states** appropriately to several of the characters in the discourse production tasks and during conversation:

Affective mental states:

> he got very *angry*
>
> (Flowerpot Incident)

> she wasn't *distressed*
>
> (Conversation)

Cognitive mental states:

> he *wants* to hold a party
>
> (Cinderella story)

> she *forgot* about the time
>
> (Cinderella story)

Pauline also displayed self-attribution of mental states, as the following examples illustrate:

> you did tell me, but I can't *remember*
> I *think* it was sheep that they had

Although Pauline could undertake relatively simple mental state attribution, she did not attribute complex intentions to any of the characters in the discourse production tasks. During the Flowerpot Incident, the man entered the building because his action was motivated by a complex intention, namely, to remonstrate with the woman who owned the apartment from which the flowerpot fell. The elderly woman gave the man's dog a bone. This action was also motivated by a complex intention, namely, to make amends for the injury that the man had sustained. In the Cookie Theft picture, the young girl **gestures** to the boy on the stool to be quiet. This gesture is motivated by a complex intention, namely, the girl wants the theft of the cookies to pass undetected. These complex intentions are consistently omitted by Pauline in her representation of these scenarios.

For the most part, Pauline made skilled use of **cohesion**, including **anaphoric reference**, **ellipsis**, and **lexical substitution** and reiteration:

Anaphoric reference:

I'm doing <u>this particular job</u>, I'm doing <u>it</u> 17 years now

Ellipsis:

it didn't happen the way it was supposed to [*happen*]

Lexical substitution:

we didn't have overshoes but then down the line we <u>did</u> [*have overshoes*]

Lexical reiteration:

it's a very rewarding <u>job</u>, I love my <u>job</u>

There were occasional lapses of cohesion, however, such as in the following extract from the Cinderella story. Pauline introduces the prince's father (i.e. the king), setting up an expectation on the part of the listener that the **pronoun** *he* refers to the king. Without warning, she then shifts the **referent** of *he* to the prince rather than the king:

the young prince's father wanted him to get married (1.21) though <u>he</u> said that he would get married if he could choose his em wife

Pauline exhibited other strengths in **pragmatics** and discourse in addition to her use of cohesion. She made appropriate use of **presupposition**, undertook repair of her utterances, and used a wide range of **deictic expressions**. The factive verb in the following utterance from the Cinderella story presupposes that Cinderella *was* the girl the prince had danced with at the ball:

Presupposition:

> the prince <u>realised</u> that was the girl he was dancing with

Pauline closely monitored her spoken output and, when necessary, initiated repair of her utterances. In this example from the Cinderella story, she uses self-initiated self-repair to correct her pronoun error:

Repair:

> when <u>she</u> got, when <u>he</u> got to Cinderella's house

Additionally, Pauline was skilled at reworking her utterances to achieve greater specificity and accuracy for the hearer, as this extract from her spontaneous conversation illustrates:

> then after three weeks, three or four weeks in, ah three and a half four weeks I'd said I'd had enough

Pauline used **deictic expressions** appropriately to relate her utterances to spatial, temporal and other features of context, as this response to an interjection from the postman reveals:

Deixis:

> I'm <u>here</u> thank you very much, do you need me to sign something?

Finally, Pauline was also adept at using **direct reported speech** in conversation such as in the following example, where she is reporting part of a conversation with her partner:

> Michael told me, he said "you did have a cough" … I'd always say "well, ah, you know I'd be wearing a mask for fifteen hours"

These pragmatic and discourse strengths alongside Pauline's reduced informativeness and poor **letter fluency** suggest some disruption of her high-level language skills that are dependent on **executive functions** such as **attention** and concentration. **Memory** may serve to exacerbate these difficulties but cannot alone account for Pauline's limited informativeness which was also evident in tasks where she had pictorial support. Further, slowed information processing may account for Pauline's self-reported word-finding difficulties in conversation and may explain her repeated use of **fillers** at critical processing junctures such as syntactic boundaries and before **noun phrases**.

COMMUNICATION PROFILE:

Speech intelligibility:

- Pauline's speech was fully intelligible. The volume, rate and fluency of her speech were in the normal range. Pauline's articulation, resonance, voice quality, breath support for speech, stress and intonation were consistent with other speakers of similar age and gender. There was no evidence of phonological impairment or motor speech disorders such as dysarthria or apraxia of speech.

Morphology and syntax:

- Pauline used a wide range of morphemes and syntactic constructions in her expressive language including prefixes, derivational and inflectional suffixes, embedded clauses and passive voice constructions. Her comprehension of these same morphemes and syntactic constructions was intact for conversation and for instructions to discourse tasks.

Vocabulary and semantics:

- Pauline displayed good confrontation naming notwithstanding reports of word-finding difficulty in conversation. Her semantic fluency scores for animals and types of fruit were consistent with normative values. Pauline made occasional use of general words (e.g. *people*) over specific words (e.g. *villagers*). Her choice of argument structure (e.g. *The door opened*) misrepresented causation and other relationships between participants in some events (e.g. *The storm ripped open the door of the barn*).

Pragmatics:

- Pauline could take turns in conversation, repair utterances and make appropriate use of linguistic politeness (e.g. her response to the postman). She used presupposition and deixis appropriately. Pauline was frequently seen to rework her utterances to fulfil expectations of specificity and accuracy on the part of the hearer.

Discourse:

- Pauline had reduced informativeness in discourse. Her informativeness was reduced relative to healthy controls and Covid controls, and occurred in contexts that were both dependent on, and independent of, memory. She ordered events correctly during narrative and procedural discourse. Pauline used a range of cohesive devices including ellipsis, lexical substitution and reiteration, and anaphoric reference. Occasionally, errors in cohesion were observed. She made skilled use of direct reported speech during conversation.

Cognition:

- Pauline had a poor letter fluency score relative to normative data, suggesting some executive function difficulties. She attributed simple cognitive and affective mental states both to her own mind and to the minds of characters in stories and pictures. She did not engage in attribution of complex intentions to these same characters. Pauline reports cognitive deficits in memory, attention and concentration since contracting Covid-19.

Suggestions for Further Reading

(1) Ramage, A.E. (2020) 'Potential for cognitive communication impairment in COVID-19 survivors: A call to action for speech-language pathologists', *American Journal of Speech-Language Pathology*, 29 (4): 1821–1832.

This is a tutorial for speech-language pathologists who are likely to play a role in the rehabilitation of cognitive-communication impairment in patients who have had Covid infection. It examines what has been reported so far about neurological insults in Covid patients. The syndrome that is most likely to resemble the cognitive deficits that may occur in Covid patients, namely, post-intensive care unit syndrome, is discussed. Finally, suggestions are provided for the cognitive-communication evaluation and intervention of Covid patients.

(2) Mohapatra, B. and Mohan, R. (2020) 'Speech-language pathologists' role in the multi-disciplinary management and rehabilitation of patients with covid-19', *Journal of Rehabilitation Medicine – Clinical Communications*, 3: 1000037. doi: 10.2340/20030711-1000037.

This article examines the role of speech-language pathologists in the management of clients with Covid-19 in acute care units, inpatient units and outpatient units. This role includes responsibility for dysphagia screening and diagnosis (acute care units), dysphagia and tracheostomy management (inpatient units), and swallowing, speech, voice and neurocognitive rehabilitation (outpatient units).

(3) Sheehy, L.M. (2020) 'Considerations for postacute rehabilitation for survivors of COVID-19', *JMIR Public Health and Surveillance*, 6 (2): e19462.

Written just over three months after SARS-CoV-2 was first reported, this article examines the rehabilitation needs, including speech-language pathology, of patients with Covid-19 after discharge from acute care. Guidelines for the management of people with long Covid, many of whom were not hospitalised (like Pauline in this case study), are currently in development: https://www.nice.org.uk/guidance/indevelopment/gid-ng10179 (National Institute for Health and Care Excellence).

Questions

(1) Pauline exhibited several pragmatic and discourse skills during conversation and other forms of discourse. What types of pragmatic and discourse skills are exemplified by the underlined parts of her utterances below?

    (a) "one of the girls who was quite poorly <u>one of my colleagues</u> (.) and em she got upset"

    (b) "the mice they got the key and <u>managed</u> to open the door"

    (c) "the wash hand <u>the sink</u> is overflowing"

    (d) "it [the swab] came back negative <u>again</u>"

    (e) "<u>these residents</u> obviously weren't ventilated some we had oxygen for some of <u>them</u> we had end-of-life medications em for <u>them</u>"

(2) Given the consistent presence of often debilitating fatigue in people with long Covid, chronic fatigue syndrome (CFS) may prove to be a model for the impact of Covid infection on language and cognition. Executive function skills have been found to be impaired in CFS,[16] but not uniformly so. Adolescents and adults with CFS have been reported to perform comparably to healthy controls on measures of cognitive flexibility (switching attention).[17,18] In the following extract from the Cinderella story, Pauline (PAR) must switch attention from her narration of the Cinderella story at the point marked '↓' to the postman who is making a delivery and then back to the narrative production task. How would you characterise her cognitive flexibility in this extract?

INV: Okay Patricia in your own time can you tell me the Cinderella story?

PAR: (3.13) Okay so (2.58) there was a young girl (1.24) who went to (1.95) she was out in the forest and she the fountain and em (.) she met this handsome young prince who was at the fountain watering his horse (1.48) then she disappeared (.) and em the young prince's father wanted him to get married (1.21) though he said that he would get married if he could choose his em wife and if he invited em he wanted to have a party to invite all the eligible young ladies in the (1.10) in the kingdom to come (1.76) and ↓ thank you (1.39) yeah I'm here thank you very much do you need me to sign something no thanks sorry it's my postman

INV: You're quite all right

PAR: So he wanted to he wants to hold a party em so invite all the young girls to come so hoping that the girl that he'd met at the fountain would end up coming to the party and he would meet her and he would be able to marry her though they invited all the eligible young ladies to the dance and em the young girl who he'd met at the fountain she had ah a stepmother and two step siser, sisters (.) so they were all invited cause they were all single they were all invited to the party but the stepsisters weren't very nice to her so they said that she couldn't …

(3) A speaker may produce under-informative discourse for several reasons. There may be information that is *omitted*. Some information may be *inaccurate* or expressed in *vague* language that conveys little meaning or content. There may be *repetition* of information that adds nothing new to the discourse. Pauline tended to produce under-informative discourse. One example was the Flowerpot Incident in which she related only 30% of the information that was essential to the story. This narrative is shown below. Give *one* example of each of the reasons just outlined why this story is less than maximally informative:

> there's a man walking down the street (1.98) and as he was walking down the street he there was bucket of water thrown out the top window (1.25) which hit him on the head he got very angry (1.21) and went up the stairs to knock on the door of the flat that had the water had come out of (.) em when the door was opened there was a beautiful lady (1.91) who gave the man and his dog a bone (.) and showed him some love and at this stage the man fell in love with the lady and they all lived happily ever after

Answers

(1) (a) Pauline revises her utterance to replace the general term *girls* with the more specific word *colleagues*, revealing an awareness on her part of hearer expectations to be as specific and informative as possible.
   (b) The implicative verb *managed* triggers a presupposition that the mice *tried* to open the door.
   (c) Pauline undertakes a self-initiated self-repair when she replaces *wash hand* with *sink*.
   (d) The iterative expression *again* triggers a presupposition that the swab came back negative *before*.
   (e) Pauline uses *them* to refer to the preceding noun phrase *these residents*. This is a form of cohesion called anaphoric reference.
(2) Pauline displays excellent cognitive flexibility during her Cinderella narration. At the point of suspending her narrative, she has conveyed two

propositions that are central to the story, namely, that a ball or party is to be held in the kingdom and that all single, young women are to be invited to it. Pauline has also related that the prince met Cinderella at the fountain. Although this is not accurate – Cinderella was at the fountain with her father, not the prince – it is a further component of the narrative that was conveyed prior to the postman's interruption. As soon as Pauline resumes her narration, she reiterates all three information elements before progressing the story. This is done with a view to ensuring that the information conveyed prior to the interruption is part of the hearer's representation of the story and has not been lost as a result of the interruption. As soon as this is achieved, Pauline is efficient at progressing the story.

(3) Pauline's Flowerpot Incident discourse is under-informative for the following reasons:

> *Omission of information*, e.g. Pauline does not state that the man is walking with his dog.
>
> *Inaccurate information*, e.g. Pauline states that the man is struck on the head by a falling bucket of water when it is, in fact, a flowerpot that strikes him.
>
> *Vague information*, e.g. Pauline states that the woman 'showed him [the man] some love'. It is not clear what this means when the actual events involve the woman giving the man's dog a bone and the man kissing the woman on the hand in gratitude.
>
> *Repeated information*, e.g. Pauline states twice that the man is walking down the street.

References

[1] Lam, T.T., Jia, N., Zhang, Y. et al. (2020) 'Identifying SARS-CoV-2 related coronaviruses in Malayan pangolins', *Nature*. doi:10.1038/s41586-020-2169-0

[2] Yang, X., Yu, Y., Xu, J. et al. (2020) 'Clinical course and outcomes of critically ill patients with SARS-CoV-2 pneumonia in Wuhan, China: A single-centered, retrospective, observational study', *Lancet Respiratory Medicine*, 8 (5): 475–481.

[3] Kimball, A., Hatfield, K.M., Arons, M., James, A., Taylor, J. et al. (2020) 'Asymptomatic and presymptomatic SARS-CoV-2 infections in residents of a long-term care skilled nursing facility – King County, Washington March 2020', *Morbidity and Mortality Weekly Report*, 69 (13): 377–381.

[4] Pan, X., Chen, D., Xia, Y., Wu, X., Li, T., Ou, X. et al. (2020) 'Asymptomatic cases in a family cluster with SARS-CoV-2 infections', *The Lancet Infectious Diseases*, 20 (4): 410–411.

[5] Chen, X., Laurent, S., Onur, O.A., Kleineberg, N.N., Fink, G.R., Schweitzer, F. and Warnke, C. (2020) 'A systematic review of neurological symptoms and complications of COVID-19', *Journal of Neurology*, doi:10.1007/s00415-020-10067-3

[6] Almeria, M., Cejudo, J.C., Sotoca, J., Deus, J. and Krupinski, J. (2020) 'Cognitive profile following COVID-19 infection: Clinical predictors leading to neuropsychological impairment', *Brain, Behavior, & Immunity – Health*, 9: 100163. doi:10.1016/j.bbih.2020.100163.

[7] Ritchie, K., Chan, D. and Watermeyer, T. (2020) 'The cognitive consequences of the COVID-19 epidemic: Collateral damage', *Brain Communications*, 2 (2): fcaa069. doi:10.1093/braincomms/fcaa069.

[8] Moss, S.E. (1995) 'Cognitive/linguistic deficits associated with chronic fatigue syndrome', *Journal of Chronic Fatigue Syndrome*, 1 (3–4): 95–100.

[9] Daly, E., Komaroff, A.L., Bloomingdale, K., Wilson, S. and Albert, M.S. (2001) 'Neuropsychological function in patients with chronic fatigue syndrome, multiple sclerosis, and depression', *Applied Neuropsychology*, 8 (1): 12–22.

[10] Park, P., Youngman, P. and Moss, S.E. (2001) 'Chronic fatigue syndrome: The role of the speech-language pathologist', *ASHA Leader*, 6 (7): 4–5, 11.

[11] Tombaugh, T.N., Kozak, J. and Rees, L. (1999) 'Normative data stratified by age and education for two measures of verbal fluency: FAS and animal naming', *Archives of Clinical Neuropsychology*, 14 (2): 167–177.

[12] Acevedo, A., Loewenstein, D.A., Barker, W.W., Harwood, D.G., Luis, C., Bravo, M., Hurwitz, D.A., Aguero, H., Greenfield, L. and Duara, R. (2000) 'Category fluency test: Normative data for English- and Spanish-speaking elderly', *Journal of the International Neuropsychological Society*, 6: 760–769.

[13] Joyce, E., Blumenthal, S. and Wesseley, S. (1996) 'Memory, attention, and executive function in chronic fatigue syndrome', *Journal of Neurology, Neurosurgery, and Psychiatry*, 60 (5): 495–503.

[14] Cvejic, E., Birch, R.C. and Vollmer-Conna, U. (2016) 'Cognitive dysfunction in chronic fatigue syndrome: A review of recent evidence', *Current Rheumatology Reports*, 18: 24. doi:10.1007/s11926-016-0577-9.

[15] Busichio, K., Tiersky, L.A., Deluca, J. and Natelson, B.H. (2004) 'Neuropsychological deficits in patients with chronic fatigue syndrome', *Journal of the International Neuropsychological Society*, 10 (2): 278–285.

[16] Santamarina-Perez, P., Eiroa-Orosa, F.J., Rodriguez-Urrutia, A., Qureshi, A. and Alegre, J. (2014) 'Neuropsychological impairment in female patients with chronic fatigue syndrome: A preliminary study', *Applied Neuropsychology: Adult*, 21 (2): 120–127.

[17] Sulheim, D., Fagermoen, E., Sivertsen, Ø.S., Winger, A., Wyller, V.B. and Øie, M.G. (2015) 'Cognitive dysfunction in adolescents with chronic fatigue: A cross-sectional study', *Archives of Disease in Childhood*, 100 (9): 838–844.

[18] Joyce, E., Blumenthal, S. and Wessely, S. (1996) 'Memory, attention, and executive function in chronic fatigue syndrome', *Journal of Neurology, Neurosurgery, and Psychiatry*, 60 (5): 495–503.

CASE STUDY 10

Guillain-Barré Syndrome

KEY FACTS AND FIGURES:

- Guillain-Barré syndrome (GBS) is an acute paralytic neuropathy that is characterised by rapidly progressive, symmetrical limb weakness with hyporeflexia or areflexia, sensory disturbances and cranial nerve deficits (in some patients).[1]
- There are clinical variants of GBS that are based on the types of nerve fibres that are involved (motor, sensory, sensory and motor, cranial or autonomic), the main mode of fibre injury (axonal versus demyelinating), and the presence of altered consciousness. Miller-Fisher syndrome (MFS) is one such variant, in which there is ophthalmoplegia, ataxia and areflexia without any weakness.[2]
- The overall incidence of GBS in the general population is between 1.1/100,000/year and 1.8/100,000/year.[3] GBS incidence increases by 20% for every 10-year increase in age.[4] A higher incidence is reported in military personnel,[5] countries with Zika virus and chikungunya virus outbreaks,[6] and women with immune disorders early in life.[7] There is a higher risk of GBS in males than in females.[4]
- Treatment for GBS involves intravenous immunoglobulin and plasma exchange. Even with current treatment, some 25% of patients require artificial ventilation, 20% are unable to walk after six months, and 3–10% of patients die.[8]
- GBS is an immune-mediated disease of the peripheral nerves and nerve roots that is typically preceded by infection. *Campylobacter jejuni* is the

DOI: 10.4324/9781003153559-11

predominant infection, accounting for 25–50% of adult cases. Other infections associated with GBS include cytomegalovirus, Epstein-Barr virus, influenza A virus, *Mycoplasma pneumoniae* and *Haemophilus influenzae*.[9] Cases of GBS have been reported in people with Covid-19 infection.[10]

- Cognitive deficits are reported in GBS.[11] Among 79 patients with GBS admitted to a neurological intensive therapy unit, 8.9% had cognitive disturbances.[12] Notwithstanding the presence of cognitive issues, the emphasis of SLP intervention in GBS is on speech, swallowing, and augmentative and alternative communication.[13–15]

Background

Carly (not her real name) is 41;8 years old. She is married and has two children aged 8 and 5 years. Carly has 21 years of formal education. She completed medical training in 2008 and paediatric residency in 2013 and is currently employed as a paediatrician. Carly works in an English- and Spanish-speaking community in the USA. English is her native language and she speaks fluent Spanish as her second language. Before pursuing a career in medicine, Carly aspired to be a civil rights attorney. Between 2000 and 2004, she held various administrative positions in law and policy but did not enjoy this work. As an undergraduate, Carly attended a women's liberal arts college where she majored in history.

In May 2020, Carly was diagnosed with the Miller-Fisher variant of GBS. This diagnosis was preceded by Covid-19 infection which had its onset on 25 March 2020. Carly's symptoms at the start of her Covid illness included fever, a burning sensation in her lungs and a dry cough. On 27 March, two days after the onset of these symptoms, Carly had a negative nasopharyngeal swab PCR test. On 17 April, she had positive IgM and IgG antibodies on the Healgen Scientific SARS-CoV-2 rapid antibody test. In late May 2020, Carly had a negative result on the SARS-CoV-2 IgG test from Quest Labs (Abbott test for nucleocapsid IgG). Carly's wife and two children developed similar symptoms 5–7 days after she became unwell. Her wife also had a positive rapid antibody test for IgM/IgG antibodies on 17 April 2020. Due to the shortage of tests, her children were never tested. Carly suspects she contracted SARS-CoV-2 through her work with sick children in a paediatric clinic in the weeks leading up to her infection. Personal protective equipment was in short supply at the start of the pandemic and many patients and their families were not wearing masks as a universal masking policy had not yet come into effect.

Carly described her health prior to Covid-19 infection as "very good". She also stated that she was "very fit and active". Her only surgical procedure to date has been a caesarean section on 17 August 2015. Carly has coeliac disease and mild ulcerative colitis which is well controlled with medication (see *Medication*). She has atopic dermatitis (eczema), hyperhidrosis (excessive sweating) and dysmenorrhoea (painful menstrual periods). She has also had gastroenteritis. Carly's hearing is normal. She has nearsightedness (myopia) which has been corrected with glasses since childhood. Carly has a normal body weight for her age, gender and height. Noteworthy features of her family history include **keratoconus**, possible **Sjögren's syndrome** and inflammatory arthritis in her mother, coeliac disease in her aunt, osteoporosis in her father and diabetes in her maternal grandparents. Carly does not smoke or vape, and she does not consume alcohol. Prior to Covid-19 infection, Carly was a competitive distance race walker. She engaged in moderate to rigorous exercise 4–5 times each week for approximately one hour at a time. Her exercise routine included weightlifting and use of the elliptical machine.

Carly eats a well-balanced diet. It is gluten free and contains minimal dairy and soy products and almost no red meat (except on holidays or at a social event). Her consumption of fish and chicken is limited. Carly eats nuts every day and fruit and vegetables. She thinks she could probably eat more vegetables, especially leafy greens. Carly has anaphylactic allergies to certain foods including peanuts and sesame. She takes several vitamin and mineral supplements. Before Covid, these supplements included vitamin D, calcium and daily fibre. As Covid cases in the USA increased, she started taking vitamin C and quercitin as well. Since her Covid illness, Carly has started taking additional supplements: alphalipoic acid, vitamin B complex, fish oil, L-glutamine and artichoke extract.

Carly reported that before her Covid illness she did not have a healthy work–life balance. She had already reduced her work hours to make more time for herself and her family but acknowledged that there was still an imbalance: "with demands placed on physicians in a customer service-driven model, where we are given no administrative time, it is impossible not to have work cut into personal time". When she did have some leisure time, Carly enjoyed race walking, hiking, camping, cooking and reading. Prior to the Covid-19 pandemic, Carly met friends socially on a regular basis. She has continued to keep in touch with her friends during the pandemic via text, phone and Zoom. She reports that the Covid online support groups have helped her to maintain connections with other people and manage her illness, which she characterises as long, slow, and involving frequent relapses and setbacks.

Carly has had several medical examinations and a hospital admission during her illness. She was hospitalised between 1 and 3 June 2020 with **tachycardia**, **ataxia**, bladder issues and difficulty with swallowing. During her stay, Carly had two chest X-rays but nothing abnormal was detected. Carly had electrocardiograms on 19 May and 1 June, and both were mildly abnormal. Her heart function was further assessed by means of echocardiograms conducted on 4 June and 6 November and the use of a Holter monitor which was worn for 30 days from 2 November. Results showed tachycardia but no **arrhythmias**. A diagnosis of **postural orthostatic tachycardia syndrome** (POTS) was confirmed, with orthostatic vitals showing pulse increase with position change and stable blood pressure. An MRI scan and **lumbar puncture** were conducted on 27 May and 1 June, respectively, and both produced normal results.

Since the onset of her Covid illness, Carly has experienced a range of visual-spatial and visual-perceptual disturbances. She reports not having depth perception. When she is in the car, she feels that cars are coming towards her. She sees things in her peripheral vision. Screens are difficult for her to tolerate. When she looks down, she can feel unbalanced. Carly was examined at the neuro-ophthalmology clinic on 21 October 2020. Her examining physician concluded, "Carly continues to suffer from a host of symptoms post-COVID. These include a number of issues often seen in the wake of general neurologic insult such as reported cognitive slowing, vestibular, visuomotor and **convergence impairment**, and **photophobia**. Prior imaging was negative and the exam today is non-localizing but the slowness of **saccade** initiation and the limitation of (e.g.) **supraduction** and also facial weakness can be seen in the setting of **Miller-Fisher Syndrome**/GBS for which she was previously empirically treated with intravenous immunoglobulin."

Carly is currently working with physical, occupational and speech therapy. Physical therapy commenced on 21 May 2020. Initial impressions suggested vestibular hypofunction and visual dependency for balance. It was also noted that Carly had hypersensitivity to visual motion and passive motion. Her occupational therapy goals are focused on increasing fine motor skills, increasing **coordination** and strength bilaterally, reducing visual deficits and returning to high-level cognition and multi-tasking. Speech therapy is targeting **working memory** and dual task **attention**. It was observed in speech therapy that Carly benefited from the re-auditorisation of sentences and extra time, and that repetition and practice increased learning and retention of information.

Clinical Symptoms

Carly's diagnosis of the Miller-Fisher variant of GBS was preceded by Covid infection, the acute phase of which was spent at home without medical supervision. Carly experienced a wide array of mostly mild to moderate symptoms during her acute illness. Among her mild symptoms were breathing difficulties, aches and pains (but only rarely), a sore throat, **conjunctivitis**, and chest pain and pressure. Her moderate symptoms included fever, coughing, gastrointestinal problems (intermittent **gastroparesis** and diarrhoea), skin rash (occasional petechial outbreaks with normal platelets) and unusual sensations (photophobia and visual processing problems). Carly also had several other moderate symptoms including **tinnitus**, insomnia, loss of appetite (but no weight loss), peripheral tingling and tachycardia. Carly had two severe symptoms during her Covid illness: fatigue and headaches. Her headaches tend to recur during flare-ups of her symptoms. Carly's fatigue is an ongoing symptom that affects her daily life.

Since developing Covid illness and Miller-Fisher variant GBS, Carly has experienced cognitive difficulties. These were assessed during a neuropsychological evaluation conducted on 24 November 2020. Based on this evaluation, she was diagnosed with mild neurocognitive impairment. Her performance in a range of cognitive domains is displayed in Table 10.1.

TABLE 10.1 Carly's performance across cognitive domains on neuropsychological evaluation

Domain	Assessment	Performance
Premorbid cognitive functioning	Advanced Clinical Systems (ACS) – Word Choice, Reliable Digit Span and Test of Premorbid Functioning (TOPF)	High average range (92nd percentile)
Memory	Test of Memory and Learning (TOMAL) selective memory test; Rey Complex Figure Test (RCFT); Wechsler Memory Scale 4th Edition (WMS-IV) logical memory subtest	*Verbal memory:* Learning on the selective list learning task on the TOMAL fell in the average range. Delayed recall of the list fell at the 75th percentile. Scores on story recall fell in the high average range for both immediate and delayed recall. Recognition of the stories fell in the high average range. Carly benefited from the structured nature of the story memory task. *Visual memory:* Recall on the RCFT fell at the 10th percentile for both immediate and delayed recall trials. Recognition fell in the average range. Carly recalled the overall gestalt of the image but forgot the details.
Attention	Paced Auditory Serial Addition Test (PASAT); Wechsler Adult Intelligence Scale, 4th Edition (WAIS-IV) digit span subtest	Carly was able to state back up to a five-digit string accurately (below average performance). Her overall digit span score fell in the below average range (16th percentile). Her performance on the PASAT, an auditory attention task, fell at the 14th percentile for Rate #1 and at the 15th percentile for Rate #2. Both scores fall in the below average range, indicating problems with complex attention tasks. Overall, a decline is seen in auditory attention tasks.

(Continued)

TABLE 10.1 (Continued)

Domain	Assessment	Performance
Visual processing	Delis-Kaplan Executive Functioning System (DKEFS) colour word subtest; Hooper Visual Object Test (HVOT)	Carly was not able to focus on tasks that were visually stimulating and had to look away. She performed poorly on tests that required her to track objects or read. Her speed for reading words and naming colours on the DKEFS colour word task fell below the 1st percentile. On the RCFT, she was able to copy the figure accurately but had difficulty in recalling details of the image. Her score on the HVOT fell at the 8th percentile, indicating difficulty with visual-spatial integration.
Executive functioning	Delis-Kaplan Executive Functioning System (DKEFS) verbal fluency test	Carly's impaired performance on the DKEFS colour word task – below the 1st percentile – is reflective of impairment with processing visual material rather than poor executive functioning. Her performance on the verbal fluency switching task of the DKEFS fell at the 75th percentile (average range).
Processing speed	Grooved Pegboard Test	Carly was slow to complete tasks. Her speed on the Grooved Pegboard Test fell below the 1st percentile for both hands. A tremor was also observed when she drew out objects.
Language	Neuropsychological Assessment Battery (NAB) naming subtest	Carly had no difficulty with confrontation naming. On the NAB naming test, she was able to name all pictures correctly. She engaged in circumlocution during the naming of *canteen*. Carly's conversational speech was fluent.

In summary, Carly's neuropsychological evaluation revealed intact performance in language, auditory memory and **executive functioning** such as **inhibition**. She had impaired performance in visual-spatial integration, visual memory, processing speed, and complex attention required for multi-tasking and dual tasks.

Carly reported experiencing **neuropsychiatric symptoms** during the first few months of her illness. When she had relapses of her physical symptoms such as chest pain, fever and chills, she had "random waves of uncontrollable emotions" that had no apparent trigger. She would cry for no reason, for example, and have waves of intense anger. As her physical symptoms improved, her neuropsychiatric symptoms also receded.

Daily Activities

Carly's Covid illness and Miller-Fisher variant GBS have had a significant impact on her daily life and activities. She has been on medical disability leave since 19 May 2020. For a once busy medical professional, the inability to work has been a stressful experience for her. Carly's ability to do household chores is very limited. She can perform sedentary tasks like folding laundry but cannot do anything that involves bending over. Before her Covid illness, Carly was very fit and undertook regular exercise. Since becoming unwell, she has only been able to do exercises recommended by her physical therapist and slow walking for 15 minutes each day. Until the end of October 2020, she was using a walker and then a cane to give her support while walking. Carly is no longer driving.

Since the onset of her illness, Carly has not been able to pursue her usual leisure activities. Activities like race walking have been replaced by LEGO building as she is now spending much more time at home with her children. Carly's cognitive difficulties have impacted her daily life. She describes how accomplishing simple tasks such as packing her son's bag for school takes much longer than normal. Carly reports decreased executive functioning. She has poor self-monitoring and problems with multi-tasking. She is trying to compensate for these difficulties with the use of lists and other strategies. Her **short-term memory** problems make it difficult for her to complete tasks that require multiple steps, such as preparing schoolwork for her child's distance learning, making a grocery list and keeping track of her many medical appointments and their various recommendations.

Medication

Carly has been taking prescribed medications related to her illness. On 18 May 2020, she was prescribed prednisone for vestibular neuritis. She took 60 mg every day for one week and smaller doses over subsequent weeks. A second course of prednisone for post-Covid inflammatory symptoms was commenced on 11 December. The dose on this occasion was 60 mg x 5 days, 40 mg x 5 days, 30 mg x 3 days, 20 mg x 3 days, 10 mg x 3 days. For acid protection while taking prednisone, Carly has taken omperazole XR 20 mg and famotidine 20 mg every day. Additionally, she has been taking famotidine 20 mg at night when needed for the treatment of **gastroesophageal reflux disease** during her **long Covid** illness. Carly has also taken Tylenol for symptom control. Two months after her initial Covid symptoms, Carly received five infusions of intravenous immunoglobulin (IVIG) for the treatment of Miller-Fisher variant GBS. Carly also takes medications that predate her Covid illness. She takes two mesalamine 1.2 g tablets daily for the treatment of ulcerative colitis. Carly also takes low-dose oestrogen oral contraceptive pills and uses an antihistamine (loratadine) for general allergies.

Communication

Carly's Covid illness and subsequent diagnosis of Miller-Fisher variant GBS have had a profound impact on her language and communication skills. She has word-finding difficulties in daily conversation and produces **semantic paraphasias** like *hairbrush* for *hairdryer*. She cannot remember the names of people she has known for a long time. Carly can have a full conversation with someone and not remember what was discussed immediately afterwards. Although she can mostly remember the topic of an ongoing conversation, she reports having moments every day where she suddenly has "no idea" what she and others are talking about. Carly can sometimes miss what someone says and then feels lost as the conversation has moved on. Her ability to read and use a computer has been limited for months on account of Covid-related visual problems. Now that she is trying to read a bit more, she has found that her comprehension of written language is very poor. She can follow simple books that she is reading to her children. Although Carly still wants to participate in conversation with others, she believes that months of limited social interaction have made conversations seem exhausting and awkward at times. Carly reports a reduction "over her baseline" in the frequency with which she communicates with others.

The author spoke to Carly online on 3 December 2020. It was 6 pm local time in the USA. The conversation lasted for 1 hour and 15 minutes. Carly was alert, responsive and cooperative throughout the session. She wore her glasses and would often look away from the computer screen as she found it difficult to tolerate it. Carly spoke in a well-lit room at home and was not disturbed by family members or others during the session. She was relaxed and spoke at ease about her Covid illness and its implications for her ability to work and undertake daily activities. She displayed no emotional distress at any point during the meeting.

Carly's speech was fully intelligible. There was no evidence of **motor speech disorder**, either **dysarthria** or **apraxia of speech**, and she did not display phonological impairment. All parameters of speech production were within the normal range for a speaker of Carly's age and gender. This included her **articulation** of speech sounds, respiratory support for speech, **resonance**, **voice quality** and **intonation**, and stress (prosody). Carly spoke fluently and had a typical speaking rate.

Carly produced well-formed utterances during her meeting with the author. She displayed intact use of inflectional morphemes, including the following **inflectional suffixes** for number, person, tense, aspect and gradation:

we couldn't test the kids at that point (*plural number −s*)
she waves her magic wand (*third-person singular −s*)

> I call<u>ed</u> my wife (*past tense –ed*)
> I was drink<u>ing</u> tons and tons of fluids (*progressive aspect –ing*)
> it was like the weird<u>est</u> sense (*gradation – superlative*)

Carly used **derivational suffixes** and prefixes consistently and accurately. The following examples are taken from her language sample:

Derivational suffixes: contag<u>ious</u>; saturat<u>ion</u>; hospital<u>ised</u>

Prefixes: <u>re</u>tested; <u>pro</u>active; <u>in</u>credibly

Carly produced and understood complex **syntax**. Her performance on the sentence generation task was 100%, showing that she could retain words in auditory memory (an area of strength for Carly) while undertaking sentence encoding. Among the complex structures that she used in her language sample were **passive voice** constructions, interrogative **subordinate clauses**, and infinitive and *that*-clauses:

> I <u>was cleared to go back to work</u>
>
> *(passive voice and infinitive clause)*

> I remember <u>I talked to my doctor</u>
>
> *(that-clause)*

> so now we dun know <u>what to do with you</u>
>
> *(non-finite interrogative subordinate clause)*

Carly had a high-level **vocabulary** and produced some words during **category fluency** tests (e.g. *sugar glider*) and **discourse** production tasks (e.g. *proclamation*) that are not part of the average lexical repertoire. This was to be expected given her educational background and professional occupation. She achieved 95% accuracy during **confrontation naming**, a finding that was consistent with her naming performance during neuropsychological evaluation. Her only error occurred when she used 'paper cup' for *thimble*. This was a visual error and may be related to the visual processing problems that Carly has experienced since her Covid illness. Notwithstanding her strong confrontation naming performance, Carly reported word-finding difficulties during conversation. These difficulties were not evident in the use of pauses and **fillers** during conversation and there were no instances of semantic paraphasia in her language sample. Although Carly struggled to name the cognitive test the speech therapist administered, she used a type of **circumlocution** – 'that really basic one' – that appeared to elicit correct naming of the Mini Mental State Examination. Carly's category fluency scores were in excess of normative values for her age, education level and gender.

She produced 31 animal names and 17 vegetable names in 60 seconds. These scores can be compared to the following published data (all figures are means):

Animal naming:[16]	Animal naming:[17]
Age (40–49 years): 20.7 names	51 cognitively normal adults: 22.0 names
Education (17–21 years): 19.5 names	*Vegetable naming:*[17]
Gender (female): 16.5 names	51 cognitively normal adults: 15.0 names

Carly's confrontation naming and category fluency performance suggest that she retains excellent skills of lexical access, retrieval and generation. However, her reports of **word-finding difficulty** cannot be disregarded and suggest that some impairment of these skills may emerge in cognitively challenging communicative contexts.

Another area where Carly's language performance was consistent with her performance during neuropsychological testing was her immediate and delayed recall of the 100-word Sam and Fred story. Carly's immediate and delayed story recall during neuropsychological testing was reported to be in the high average range. Carly recalled 71% of the essential information units in the Sam and Fred story, with no deterioration in her performance between immediate and delayed recall. Carly lost marks on this task when she used general words and expressions in place of more specific linguistic expressions used in the story. Examples of her recall are shown below, with words on the right of the arrow replacing those that were used in the story (shown on left of arrow):

sheep and cows → 'animals'

door of the barn was ripped open → 'damage barn'

sheep and cows were returned to the barn → 'animals back in'

storm → 'big huge rain flood-like thing'

In terms of **semantics**, Carly produced meaningful sentences that expressed a wide range of conceptual relations between events. The conjunctions in the following sentences express meanings of consequence, condition, reason and time between the **clauses** that they conjoin:

we were low on swabs <u>so</u> they couldn't, you couldn't get retested

(*consequence*)

<u>if</u> our country could just get it together and we would have like this universal thing, it would be great

(*condition*)

the stepmother and stepdaughter um don't like Cinderella <u>because</u> she's
beautiful and kind

(reason)

that actually got better pretty quick <u>after</u> I got by the IVIG

(time)

Carly also used a range of **semantic roles** to represent participants and events
in **discourse**. This included **agent**, patient, goal, source and location, as the following utterances illustrate:

the brother [AGENT] has climbed up on a stool [GOAL]
a potted plant [PATIENT] falls off of a balcony [SOURCE]
she [AGENT] locks Cinderella [PATIENT] in her shed [LOCATION]

Carly displayed many pragmatic language skills. She delivered an informative
account of her Covid illness over a period of several months. Her narrative was
skillfully sequenced according to the timing of her symptoms and medical investigations and was unaided by any written record of these events. Carly's account
of her illness suggested a speaker who was aware of her listener's knowledge state
(an important **theory of mind** skill) and was able to structure her account to
ensure maximal comprehension on the part of her listener. One area that was
noteworthy was Carly's use of hedges such as *sort of* and *kind of*:

I got exposed at work am and then I developed you know **sort of** a first
couple days **sort of** a scratchy throat and a dry cough and **kind of** a low-
grade fever

Hedges occurred with high frequency during Carly's account of her illness.
There were 18 instances of *sort of* alone when she described her symptoms. The
symptoms of Covid illness were often unclear, even to those with the infection,
and this high frequency of **hedging** may reflect this lack of certainty. Also, Carly
was attempting to recall from **memory** a complex set of events during a stressful
time for her and her family. Her use of hedging may signify a lack of clear recall
of these events. Of course, hedging is a pragmatic device that speakers use when
they want to modify their epistemic commitment to a claim – Carly could not
recall her symptoms with certainty because they were rather vague and non-
specific in nature, some time had elapsed since she experienced them, and so
on. Carly's extensive use of hedging reveals that she is attentive to the veracity
of her utterances. Carly also extensively reworked her utterances to ensure their
accuracy for the hearer. In the following extract, she is trying to be as specific as
possible about the restrictions that were in force in her area:

we were under a, so our Governor went in, put us into lockdown, am not
lockdown I guess they call it 'shelter in place' but same deal

Carly fulfilled conversational expectations to be accurate and informative in the utterances that she produced. She was able to do this ultimately because she understood the mental states of her hearer, and particularly what her hearer already *knew* (and, by implication, what her listener needed to be told). Mental state attribution or **theory of mind** is integral to **utterance interpretation**.[18–21] Carly was also skilled at attributing mental states to the characters in stories and other discourse production tasks. The following utterances illustrate her use of both cognitive and **affective mental state** language. The final example also illustrates the self-attribution of a mental state (Carly attributes a cognitive mental state to her own mind):

they were <u>thinking</u> the weather was going to change

(cognitive mental state)

the man becomes very <u>angry</u>

(affective mental state)

she's <u>sad</u> and alone

(affective mental state)

the prince <u>wants</u> to have every young lady see ...

(cognitive mental state)

the dog is <u>happy</u>, so I <u>guess</u> the guy is over it

(affective and cognitive mental states)

Other aspects of **pragmatics** used appropriately in Carly's expressive language were **idioms, presuppositions** and **deixis**. The change-of-state verb *started* in the second example below triggers the presupposition that Carly had not felt tired before. In the final example, the neurologist who is reported to have asked Carly to *come* into the office locates Carly at a distance from the reported speaker with movement towards that speaker. Carly is skilled at representing her distal relationship to the reported speaker through her use of spatial deixis:

my son like never wants to do Spanish so like he <u>hit the jackpot</u>

(idiom)

I sort of <u>started</u> feeling super tired

(presupposition)

I'm with the neurologist over video and she's like "how soon could you <u>come</u> into the office"

(spatial deixis)

The final example above is important in a further regard. Carly made extensive use of reported speech in her account of her Covid illness. She weaved her way seamlessly between the reported utterances of medical professionals as she recounted the symptoms of her illness. Reported speech is a complex pragmatic language skill that Carly employed to good effect in conversational discourse:

> they said **"great, you don't have Covid"** and I said **"ok, cool, I'm glad"** but you know as kind of the disease progressed and seemed to follow very ah (1.03) textbook-like Covid description you know the you know within a week feeling like very short of breath then being very dizzy and developing **tachycardia** worse with movement then my oxygen saturation dropping but never really below the sort of low to mid-nineties severe insomnia am body aches chills yeah am I was sort of like **"hum, you sure I don't have Covid"** (*laughter*)

Carly used **cohesive devices** to good effect in conversation and other forms of **discourse**. She used the **demonstrative pronoun** *this* and the **adverb** *there* to link utterances through **anaphoric reference**:

> I have this weird sort of slightly abnormal <u>EKG</u> but then the cardiologist said "oh no, it's fine, don't worry about it, it was a machine error" like who knows, I don't really, I don't really do <u>this</u> in paediatrics
>
> (*anaphoric 'this'*)

> I got sent to a <u>speech therapist</u> about um (1.15) after Guillain-Barré so now, where are we now, we're in er, we're in early July right (.) and I was sent <u>there</u> for the swallowing problems
>
> (*anaphoric 'there'*)

Other cohesive devices that contributed to the comprehensibility of Carly's discourse were **lexical substitution** and **ellipsis**:

> she [the speech therapist] was just doing her intakes "oh, let me give you a <u>cognitive test</u>" right, right, um so she gives me whatever, like the what is it called, the MMSE, I mean that really basic <u>one</u>, Mini Mental Status Examination
>
> (*lexical substitution*)

> I mean there was urgency but there wasn't [urgency] and a lot was unknown, and a lot was missing
>
> (*ellipsis*)

Notwithstanding these various discourse strengths, Carly tended to omit information from discourse. Her most informative discourse was the Flowerpot Incident, in which she produced 75% of key information. However, this was little more informative than her immediate and delayed recall of the Sam and Fred story, where she produced 71% of key information and had to rely on auditory memory only (an area of strength for Carly). Her other two discourse production tasks – the Cookie Theft picture description task and the Cinderella narration – were less informative still, with Carly conveying only 67% and 66% of key information, respectively. The pictorial support provided by these tasks appeared not to increase the informativeness of the discourse that Carly produced. This is consistent with the finding of Carly's neuropsychological evaluation that visual aspects of cognition, namely, visual memory and visual-spatial integration, were areas of impairment for her.

In her description of the Cookie Theft picture, Carly's visual difficulties are apparent. She omitted that the mother was standing in a puddle of water, and that the girl had her arm outstretched to receive a cookie and was gesturing to her brother to be quiet. These less salient details require her to have visually scanned the entire scene. Meanwhile, Carly states incorrectly that an animal is outside the window. Also, despite acknowledging that it is "odd" that the mother does not notice all these activities going on around her, Carly does not attribute to the mother a mental state that might explain her neglect, namely, that she is daydreaming or is otherwise distracted. The latter **inference** requires her to examine the mother's vacant facial expression, another aspect of the description that may be compromised by Carly's visual processing problems:

Cookie Theft:

> okay so there's a mom (1.18) I'm assuming she's a mom who looks like she's tryin' to wash her dishes but then her sink is overflowing um and then like (.) while that's going on the brother has climbed up on a stool to sneak out a cookie so he's tryin' to hand a cookie to sister and he's about to fall off the stool (1.57) um (.) and then (.) outside I (2.69) I think that's a bush but at first I once again my eyes played a lot of tricks on me like is that something is that like an animal outside their window (1.42) but I think it's yeah um so (1.21) yeah (.) um it is sort of odd the whole thing because the woman looks like a total nineteen fifties like everything's perfect housewife and not noticing like all these issues goin' on

Finally, Carly obtained a **letter fluency** score of 31 words beginning F, A and S in 60 seconds. She produced 11 'F' words, 10 'A' words and 10 'S' words in 60 seconds. This places her well below normative scores on letter fluency for her age, education level and gender based on published studies (all figures are means):

Letter fluency:[16]	Letter fluency:[17]
Age (40–49 years): 43.5 words	Letter 'F': 16.8 words
Education (17–21 years): 43.9 words	Letter 'A': 15.6 words
Gender (female): 37.8 words	Letter 'S': 16.9 words

Although Carly performed well on the **inhibition** component of **executive functioning** during her neuropsychological evaluation, her poor letter fluency score suggests that not all aspects of executive functioning are in the normal range. Carly's processing speed for the performance of tasks is reduced, a feature observed during her neuropsychological evaluation and reported by Carly in her daily activities. Reduced processing speed may be playing a role in Carly's poor letter fluency performance. Such executive function limitations as Carly's letter fluency performance reveals may explain some of her difficulties in integrating visual information within a maximally informative description of the Cookie Theft picture.

Carly's illness has had a particularly severe impact on her ability to communicate in Spanish, her second language. She reports that all the difficulties she is experiencing in English are also present in Spanish only they are "much worse" in Spanish. In the early months of her illness, she could not follow a simple conversation in Spanish even though she was previously fluent in the language. Her comprehension of Spanish has improved slightly but is still nowhere close to its premorbid level.

COMMUNICATION PROFILE:

Speech intelligibility:

- Carly's speech was fully intelligible. All aspects of speech production, including articulation, resonance, phonation, prosody, and respiration, were in the normal range for a speaker of Carly's age and gender. Carly's speech rate and fluency were unremarkable. She had no motor speech disorder or phonological impairment.

Morphology and syntax:

- Carly's utterances were well-formed and structurally complex. She used an extensive range of prefixes and derivational and inflectional suffixes. Carly used complex syntax including finite and non-finite clauses, passive voice constructions and subject-auxiliary inversion for questions (e.g. "Do you want me to grab the notes I took?"). Carly's comprehension of syntax was also an area of strength based on her understanding of the author's instructions and questions.

Vocabulary and semantics:

- Carly reports word-finding difficulties in conversation, although this was not apparent in her language sample. Her confrontation naming performance was very strong. Her only error in confrontation naming was visual in nature. There were no instances of semantic paraphasia in her language sample and only one possible circumlocution. Carly's category fluency scores for animals and vegetables exceeded normative values for people of the same age, education level and gender. Carly produced meaningful utterances. She expressed complex conceptual relations in the utterances she produced and used a range of semantic roles to represent participants and events.

Pragmatics:

- Carly's pragmatic language skills included the use of presuppositions, idioms and deixis. She used hedging extensively to modify her epistemic commitment to statements, especially when they related to her illness and symptoms. Carly's utterances in conversation were informative and relevant. She was aware of conversational expectations to be accurate and specific, and reworked utterances to fulfil these expectations. Carly made appropriate use of humour and laughter.

Discourse:

- Carly used a range of cohesive devices, including ellipsis, lexical substitution and anaphoric reference, to link utterances in discourse. She used reported speech extensively as she recounted events during her illness. Carly omitted information from discourse when this required her to scan and process visual information in pictures. She was able to plan and sequence events in a narrative and steps in everyday tasks.

Cognition:

- Neuropsychological evaluation revealed that verbal (auditory) memory was an area of strength for Carly, as evidenced by her high average performance on immediate and delayed story recall. Evaluation also revealed strengths in inhibition, although Carly's impaired performance on letter fluency tasks suggested other aspects of executive functioning were impaired. Impaired performance was reported in visual-spatial integration, visual memory, processing speed and complex attention. Carly displayed theory of mind skills. She attributed cognitive and affective mental states to the characters in stories, even if not on all occasions where this was warranted. When Carly was required to process visual information in pictures, her attribution of mental states was somewhat less efficient.

Suggestions for Further Reading

(1) Stoltenberg, C. (2018) 'Behind the ventilator: An SLP finds her voice as a patient with Guillain-Barré syndrome', *The ASHA Leader*, 23 (9). doi: 10.1044/leader.FPLP.23092018.72.

Carly Stoltenberg, a 46-year-old speech-language pathologist with 23 years of clinical experience, relates her experience of being completely paralysed and dependent on a ventilator as a result of developing Guillain-Barré syndrome. From this rare personal perspective, Carly offers several insights that can help speech-language pathologists in their assessment and treatment of clients with GBS.

(2) Willison, H.J., Jacobs, B.C. and van Doorn, P.A. (2016) 'Guillain-Barré syndrome', *Lancet*, 388: 717–727.

This seminar provides a comprehensive and accessible medical overview of Guillain-Barré syndrome. It examines epidemiology, pathophysiology, classification and variants of GBS, and is an ideal primer for speech-language pathologists who are coming to the assessment and treatment of this disorder for the first time.

(3) Marshall, S. and Hurtig, R.R. (2019) 'Developing a culture of successful communication in acute care settings: Part I. Solving patient-specific issues', *Perspectives of the ASHA Special Interest Groups*, 4 (5): 1028–1036.

This article contains a case study of a 28-year-old man called Jason with Guillain-Barré syndrome. Jason had total body paralysis requiring prolonged ventilation. He spent four months in hospital, two of which were in an intensive care unit. The case study examines how Jason's only reliable gesture, a very slight head tilt to the right side, became integral to his AAC intervention, and how Jason increasingly advocated for himself and his communication needs during his hospital stay.

Questions

(1) Carly used a range of pragmatic and discourse skills. Some of these skills are illustrated by the utterances below. Match each of the underlined elements in these utterances to one of the following skills: *idiom – presupposition – anaphoric reference – repair – hedge*

(a) "then her father dies and then (.) <u>um or wait I'm sorry then the mother dies</u>"

(b) "I called <u>the doctor</u> I mean <u>she's</u> just like <u>she's</u> like wait what test"

(c) "I was <u>sort of</u> starting to feel a bit better"

(d) "my ears had <u>started</u> ringing by this point"

(e) "not that I want <u>to throw anyone under the bus</u>"

(2) Carly's neuropsychological evaluation revealed problems with visual aspects of cognition. In Carly's language sample, these difficulties were most evident when she was required to integrate visual information from a pictured scene into a narrative or description. During the Cookie Theft picture description task, Carly omitted information where this required her to attend to less visually salient parts of the picture. In the following Flowerpot Incident narrative, Carly omits some essential information, thereby reducing the informativeness of her story telling. What key information does she omit?

Flowerpot Incident:

> alright so guy's out walking his dog when a plant in a, a potted plant I guess yeah that's the right word falls off of a balcony (.) um (.) and the man becomes very angry so he's like shaking his cane and probably saying some not nice things and the dog is barking um and then he actually enters the apartment building goes up the stairs and bangs on the door (.) at which point a woman opens the, the door with a bone for the dog and then (1.07) the dog is happy so I guess the guy is over it and kisses her hand as they are about to leave

(3) Carly was a skilled narrator. Her narration of the Cinderella story was well organised, informative and accurate. Her narrative is shown in full below. Examine it in detail and then answer the following questions:

Cinderella story:

> so once upon a time there's a girl named Cinderella who (.) lives with her father and has a normal happy life and then her father dies and then (.) um or wait I'm sorry then the mother dies so then the father

remarries an evil stepmother who has two daughters of her own (.) and they become her evil stepsisters so the stepmother and stepdaughter um don't like Cinderella because she's beautiful and kind and they're super jealous so then they basically um (.) turn her into like a, a maid then she has to sis, sis, slave away for them and she doesn't she makes friends with the animals um (1.39) and the sis the sis stepsisters I guess are really um, um mean and bratty so I don't think (.) the animals like them very much um so then one day the I guess they send a messenger that there's going to be a ball um and the proclamation is being read and Cinderella like hears this so she runs to her little like ah shed that she lives in and like the like the animals I think find her like awh the, the stuff and they make her a dress but then the evil stepmother and stepsisters see it and they tear it off and they tell her like she's not going and the evil stepmom takes the stepsisters to the ball (.) so (1.39) then she's sad and alone but then the, the fairy godmother comes and ah (1.28) says don't worry sweetie I'll hook you up (laughter) and she turns a pumpkin into a coach and the mice turn into like (.) white horses and then she waves her magic wand and Cinderella has like a ball gown an two glass slippers (.) and she says go on have fun but like you, you'd better be back by midnight don't stay past midnight so she goes to the ball in her (.) coach whatever and then um (1.32) the prince sees her and I guess it's like love at first sight and then they're dancing the night away and she doesn't realise the time and then she hears the clock start to strike twelve right so she's like dashing down the stairs to try to get away and she like loses one of the slippers and then I guess she yeah she gets away but then the coach turns back into a pumpkin and then she's back in her rags (.) and so then I guess that day or the next day whatever the, the kingdom is a buzz and there was another messenger because the prince wants to have every one young lady see if their foot fits the glass slipper and the stepmom is so worried she locks Cinderella in her shed but the mice steal the key and let her out and she tries the slipper on just in time and it fits and then they take her away to the palace to meet her prince and they get married and live happily ever after

(a) One of the reasons why Carly's narrative is so easy to follow is that she makes skilled use of cohesive devices like anaphoric reference. On one occasion, however, her use of anaphoric reference breaks down when she uses a personal pronoun that lacks a clear referent. Identify where this occurs in the narrative.

(b) Carly's skills as a narrator are reflected in her effective use of direct reported speech. Where does Carly use this speech in her narrative?

(c) Carly observes two conventions on the telling of a fairy tale, a type of fictional narrative. Where do these conventions occur?

(d) As well as not knowing who sent a messenger, there is a further reason why a listener might struggle to integrate the ball into the story. What is that reason?

(e) What feature of Carly's narrative indicates that she is closely monitoring her spoken output, an important executive function skill?

Answers

(1) (a) repair

(b) anaphoric reference

(c) hedge

(d) presupposition

(e) idiom

(2) Carly omits the key event in the story, namely, that the falling flowerpot *strikes* the man on the head. This omission appears to be related to her concern to identify accurately the type of plant that fell off the balcony. Some other information is also omitted. For example, on hearing that the man "bangs on the door", we might reasonably ask *of what*? Also, although Carly states that the man is very angry, there is no mention of any of the other mental states or complex intentions that are motivating the actions of the characters, e.g. that the man wants to remonstrate with the owner of the apartment (this is *why* he enters the building) and that the woman wants to make amends for the injury the man has sustained (this is *why* the woman gives the man's dog a bone).

(3) (a) Carly states in her narrative "they send a messenger". However, there is no prior referent for the pronoun *they* in the wider discourse context.

(b) Carly uses direct reported speech when she introduces the fairy god-mother into her story telling:

the fairy godmother comes and ah (1.28) says **"don't worry sweetie I'll hook you up"**
she says **"go on have fun but like you, you'd better be back by midnight don't stay past midnight"**

(c) Carly opens the fairy tale with the words "once upon a time" and closes it with the words "they live happily ever after".

(d) Carly provides no account of why the ball takes place, namely, that the elderly king wants his son, the prince, to find a suitable woman to marry and provide an heir to the throne.

(e) At the start of Carly's narrative, she commits an error when she states that Cinderella's father is the first of her parents to die (it is, in fact, her mother who dies first). Carly displays good error monitoring and quickly moves to correct her mistake.

References

[1] van den Berg, B., Walgaard, C., Drenthen, J., Fokke, C., Jacobs, B.C. and van Doorn, P.A. (2014) 'Guillain-Barré syndrome: Pathogenesis, diagnosis, treatment and prognosis', *Nature Reviews Neurology*, 10: 469–482.

[2] Dimachkie, M.M. and Barohn, R.J. (2013) 'Guillain-Barré syndrome and variants', *Neurologic Clinics*, 31 (2): 491–510.

[3] McGrogan, A., Madle, G.C., Seaman, H.E. and de Vries, C.S. (2009) 'The epidemiology of Guillain-Barré syndrome worldwide: A systematic literature review', *Neuroepidemiology*, 32 (2): 150–163.

[4] Sejvar, J.J., Baughman, A.L., Wise, M. and Morgan, O.W. (2011) 'Population incidence of Guillain-Barré syndrome: A systematic review and meta-analysis', *Neuroepidemiology*, 36 (2): 123–133.

[5] Nelson, L., Gormley, R., Riddle, M.S. et al. (2009) 'The epidemiology of Guillain-Barré syndrome in U.S. military personnel: A case-control study', *BMC Research Notes*, 2, 171. doi:10.1186/1756-0500-2-171

[6] Capasso, A., Ompad, D.C., Vieira, D.L., Wilder-Smith, A. and Tozan, Y. (2019) 'Incidence of Guillain-Barré syndrome (GBS) in Latin America and the Caribbean before and during the 2015–2016 Zika virus epidemic: A systematic review and meta-analysis', *PLoS Neglected Tropical Diseases*, 13 (8): e0007622. doi:10.1371/journal.pntd.0007622

[7] Auger, N., Quach, C., Healy-Profitós, J., Dinh, T. and Chassé, M. (2018) 'Early predictors of Guillain-Barré syndrome in the life course of women', *International Journal of Epidemiology*, 47 (1): 280–288.

[8] van Doorn, P.A. (2013) 'Diagnosis, treatment and prognosis of Guillain-Barré syndrome (GBS)', *Presse Medicale*, 42 (6 Pt 2): e193–e201. doi:10.1016/j.lpm.2013.02.328.

[9] Willison, H.J., Jacobs, B.C. and van Doorn, P.A. (2016) 'Guillain-Barré syndrome', *Lancet*, 388: 717–727.

[10] Caress, J.B., Castoro, R.J., Simmons, Z., Scelsa, S.N., Lewis, R.A., Ahlawat, A. and Narayanaswami, P. (2020) 'COVID-19-associated Guillain-Barré syndrome: The early pandemic experience', *Muscle & Nerve*, 62 (4): 485–491.

[11] Rougé, A., Lemarié, J., Gibot, S. and Bollaert, P.E. (2016) 'Long-term impact after fulminant Guillain-Barré syndrome, case report and literature review', *International Medical Case Reports Journal*, 9, 357–363. doi:10.2147/IMCRJ.S112050

[12] Ng, K.K.P., Howard, R.S., Fish, D.R., Hirsch, N.P., Wiles, C.M., Murray, N.M.F. and Miller, D.H. (1995) 'Management and outcome of severe Guillain-Barré syndrome', *QJM: An International Journal of Medicine*, 88 (4): 243–250.

[13] Kazandjian, M. and Dikeman, K. (2012) 'Guillain-Barré syndrome and disordered swallowing', *Perspectives on Swallowing and Swallowing Disorders*, 21 (4): 115–120.

[14] Dietrich-Burns, K., Lewis, W.J.B., Lesley, D.Y. and Solomon, N.P. (2013) 'Silent aspiration and recovery from dysphagia in a case of Bickerstaff brainstem encephalitis', *Military Medicine*, 178 (1): e121–e124.

[15] Fried-Oken, M., Howard, J.M. and Stewart, S.R. (1991) 'Feedback on AAC intervention from adults who are temporarily unable to speak', *Augmentative and Alternative Communication*, 7 (1): 43–50.

[16] Tombaugh, T.N., Kozak, J. and Rees, L. (1999) 'Normative data stratified by age and education for two measures of verbal fluency: FAS and animal naming', *Archives of Clinical Neuropsychology*, 14 (2): 167–177.

[17] Clark, D.G., McLaughlin, P.M., Woo, E., Hwang, K., Hurtz, S., Ramirez, L., Eastman, J., Dukes, R.-M., Kapur, P., DeRamus, T.P. and Apostolova, L.G. (2016) 'Novel verbal fluency scores and structural brain imaging for prediction of cognitive outcome in mild cognitive impairment', *Alzheimer's & Dementia: Diagnosis, Assessment & Disease Monitoring*, 2: 113–122.

[18] Cummings, L. (2013) 'Clinical pragmatics and theory of mind', in A. Capone, F. Lo Piparo & M. Carapezza (eds), *Perspectives on Linguistic Pragmatics*, Series: Perspectives in Pragmatics, Philosophy & Psychology, Vol. 2. Cham, Switzerland: Springer International Publishing AG, 23–56.

[19] Cummings, L. (2014) 'Pragmatic disorders and theory of mind', in L. Cummings (ed.) *Cambridge Handbook of Communication Disorders*. Cambridge: Cambridge University Press, 559–577.

[20] Cummings, L. (2015) 'Theory of mind in utterance interpretation: The case from clinical pragmatics', *Frontiers in Psychology*, 6: 1286. doi:10.3389/fpsyg.2015.01286

[21] Cummings, L. (2017) 'Cognitive aspects of pragmatic disorders', in L. Cummings (ed.), *Research in Clinical Pragmatics*, Series: Perspectives in Pragmatics, Philosophy & Psychology, Vol. 11. Cham, Switzerland: Springer International Publishing AG, 587–616.

[22] Cummings, L. (2016) 'Reported speech: A clinical pragmatic perspective', in A. Capone, F. Kiefer & F. Lo Piparo (eds), *Indirect Reports and Pragmatics*, Series: Perspectives in Pragmatics, Philosophy & Psychology, Vol. 5. Cham, Switzerland: Springer International Publishing AG, 31–55.

CONCLUSION

In the Introduction to this volume, several questions were posed. For convenience, they are repeated below:

-   To what extent are impairments of language in adults with neurodegenerative disorders related to deficits in linguistic structure?
-   To what extent are impairments of language in adults with neurodegenerative disorders related to diagnosed or self-reported cognitive deficits?
-   Are language impairments present in adults with neurodegenerative disorders even in the absence of dementia or cognitive impairment?
-   Are adults with neurodegenerative disorders adept at compensating for their speech and language impairments?
-   Do impaired and preserved language skills sit alongside each other, even within the same level of language?
-   Do adults with neurodegenerative disorders exhibit impairments of linguistic competence, communicative competence, or both?
-   Do conversational partners facilitate or dominate exchanges with adults who have neurodegenerative disorders?

To draw conclusions or lessons from the case studies in this volume, each of these questions will be addressed in turn. Language samples and literature will be used to support the conclusions so drawn.

DOI: 10.4324/9781003153559-12

Are Language Impairments Related to Deficits in Linguistic Structure?

With respect to linguistic structure, the case studies in this volume reveal considerable consistency among individuals with **neurodegenerative disorders** – **morphology** and **syntax** are relatively intact even as there are considerable impairments in other levels of language. This is true of the receptive *and* expressive use of morphological and syntactic structures. From this pattern of impairment, we can conclude that where individuals display deficits in high-level language such as **pragmatics** and **discourse**, it is generally *not* the case that these deficits are related to a lack of linguistic structures. In other words, most individuals with neurodegenerative disorders had the syntactic resources needed to form **speech acts**, represent shared knowledge in the **presuppositions** of an utterance, and contribute informative, relevant utterances to conversation.

There were only two individuals where this was not so clearly the case – the man with CBD in case study 1 and the woman with HD in case study 3. Although the man with CBD was able to produce some well-formed utterances, he also produced many utterances with omitted words and grammatical errors. The woman with HD displayed some incomplete syntactic structure. However, she was also able to use a range of syntactic structures, including relative and **infinitive clauses**, **passive voice** constructions, negation and **topicalisation**. This is consistent with the findings of studies that have investigated syntax in people with HD. These studies have found that patients with HD produce high rates of syntactic errors, and a reduced number of utterances and well-formed sentences without a reduction of syntactic complexity, measured by the number of dependent clauses.[1] Notwithstanding their syntactic impairments, even these adults with neurodegenerative disorders had sufficient grammatical structures for high-level language use.

Although grammatical structure was relatively well preserved, the same was not true of the lexical abilities of several adults with neurodegeneration in these case studies. Individuals with CBD, PSP and HD displayed the most marked lexical difficulties. **Lexical retrieval** deficits were apparent for some participants during **confrontation naming**. Even when confrontation-naming performance was relatively intact, individual participants displayed word-finding difficulties in conversation. **Cueing** strategies were often, but not always, successful in eliciting production of target words during confrontation naming. Cues were semantic, phonemic, orthographic and gestural in nature. When lexical errors arose, they were most often semantic in nature – the adult with neurodegeneration produced a word that was semantically related to the target word (e.g. the adult with HD who named a seahorse as *dolphin*). Other lexical errors were visual in nature in that they bore a visual resemblance to a target word (e.g. the adult with ARBD who named an artichoke as *pineapple*). **Circumlocutions** arose infrequently, such as when the adult with CBD said "the weather came down" for *raining*. **Neologisms** were not a feature of language use in the adults in these case studies. When word-finding difficulties occurred in conversation, they were indicated by the presence of micro-pauses, often before **content words**, the use of **fillers** like *um* and *eh*, and reliance on empty words like *stuff* and *things*.

It was individuals with CBD, PSP and HD who displayed the most marked lexical-semantic impairments in these case studies. There is some support for these impairments in the published literature. Confrontation naming is impaired in some patients with CBD but often only mildly so.[2] Lexical-semantic deficits have been reported in non-clinically aphasic participants with PSP.[3] Patients with PSP have been found to perform significantly worse than controls on lexical-semantic tasks, with lower performance observed on oral and written naming, and auditory and visual comprehension of action-verbs compared to nouns.[4] Findings of lexical-semantic impairment in HD are less conclusive. While some studies have reported difficulty on lexico-semantic tasks and in retrieving the lexical forms of nouns,[5,6] other investigations indicate that people with HD are unimpaired at the lexico-semantic level.[1,7] It is noteworthy that the individuals with CBD, PSP and HD also had some of the worst **category fluency** scores across the case studies. Category fluency is a test of lexical generation. The category fluency scores of the participants with CBD and PSP were reduced relative to healthy participants but consistent with those of clinical subjects. However, the woman with HD had a category fluency score that placed her below not only healthy participants but also clinical subjects. The only other participant with such a poor category fluency score was the man with MND in case study 7.

Based on our case studies, we can say that grammatical structure (morphology and syntax) was an area of relative strength in the adults with neurodegeneration. Although impaired in some participants, lexical-semantic abilities were not sufficiently disrupted to account for the types of high-level language impairments seen in these adults. So, in answer to our question, language impairments were not entirely, or even mostly, related to deficits in linguistic structure. But there is a further conclusion that we can draw. The relative sparing of the grammatical structure of language alongside disruption of the mental lexicon is consistent with reports of language impairment in neurodegeneration in the literature. It is now widely acknowledged that language levels deteriorate at different stages of neurodegeneration, with semantic and pragmatic deficits evident quite early in the disease course, and phonological and syntactic skills often last to be disrupted (at least in **Alzheimer's disease**).[8] This appears to be borne out by the findings of relatively intact **syntax** and mild to moderate lexical-semantic impairment in several of the subjects in these case studies.

Are Language Impairments Related to Diagnosed or Self-Reported Cognitive Deficits?

Cognitive impairment in the absence of **dementia** was either diagnosed or self-reported in nearly all subjects in these case studies. An exception was the man with MND in case study 7 who reported that he had normal cognitive skills "for someone of his age". Four subjects had received formal assessment of their cognitive skills. They were the individuals with CBD, LBD, ARBD and **Guillain-Barré syndrome** in case studies 1, 4, 8 and 10, respectively. The subject with CBD in case study 1 was extensively assessed using a range of cognitive tests: Folstein Mini-Mental State Examination (MMSE); Addenbrooke's Cognitive Examination Revised (ACE-R); Wechsler Memory Scale Fourth Edition; Wechsler Adult Intelligence Scale Fourth Edition (WAIS-IV); and Delis Kaplan Executive Function System. Early assessment using the Folstein Mini-Mental State Examination revealed no cognitive impairment. However, as the subject's condition progressed and other cognitive assessments were performed, deficits in processing speed, **attention**, language and **memory** were identified. The Montreal Cognitive Assessment (MoCA) and the ACE-R (incorporating the MMSE) were used to assess the man with LBD in case study 4. The MoCA was used on several occasions to examine the man with ARBD in case study 8. When the MoCA was first administered during an extended hospital admission, it revealed that this individual had moderate cognitive impairment. With subsequent administration, cognitive performance returned to normal. Although this performance undoubtedly reflected an improvement in the patient's medical condition and cognitive status, practice effects from the repeated use of the test could not be excluded.

Because results from formal cognitive assessments were not available for all participants, phonemic (letter) fluency scores were recorded for all case study participants. As expected, nearly all participants obtained **phonemic fluency** scores that were lower than normative scores for healthy participants. The single exception was the man with MND in case study 7 whose phonemic fluency score was consistent with that of healthy participants. Additionally, nearly all participants obtained phonemic fluency scores that were either consistent with, or lower than, normative values for individuals with neurodegenerative disorders. The two exceptions were case studies 1 and 7 where the participants with CBD and MND, respectively, obtained phonemic fluency scores that were higher than normative values for individuals with these neurodegenerative disorders. Poor phonemic fluency performance indicates that there are problems with **executive functioning** in most individuals with neurodegeneration in these case studies and supports assessment findings and self-reports of cognitive impairment in these study participants. The issue, then, is the extent to which cognitive impairment contributes to the language difficulties of these case-study participants.

The generation, **planning** and execution of **discourse** in tasks such as story-telling require the integration of executive function skills. When these skills are impaired or are poorly integrated in individuals with neurodegeneration, discourse may be repetitive and under-informative, information may be conveyed in the wrong order, and digression may occur. Events in a story may be poorly related to each other (local connectedness) and to the theme or purpose of a narrative (global connectedness). It may be difficult for adults with neurodegeneration and **executive dysfunction** to convey the gist of a narrative and the lesson or moral of a story. These discourse anomalies are well evidenced in the literature. Patients with CBD make less reference to the theme of a narrative and display poorer global and local connectedness than healthy participants.[9] Individuals with **Parkinson's disease** exhibit reduced cohesive adequacy in **narrative discourse**, evidenced by a high percentage of incomplete and erroneous cohesive ties.[10] Patients with Lewy body dementia have significant difficulty organising narrative speech. Moreover, this narrative impairment is correlated with deficits on measures of executive functioning.[11]

These same discourse problems were evident in the adults with neurodegeneration in the case studies. The adult with CBD in case study 1 retained knowledge of narrative structure. However, he omitted, repeated and incorrectly sequenced information and sometimes used **cohesive devices** inaccurately. He also sometimes drew erroneous **inferences** from visual information when telling a story based on pictures. In case study 3, the woman with HD repeated and omitted information in discourse and conveyed contradictory information. She was, however, able to use **ellipsis** and **pronominal reference** effectively as cohesive devices. The woman with MS in case study 5 also made effective use of **cohesion** in discourse. However, she often drew mistaken inferences from pictures, leading to misinterpretation of events. She also omitted information from discourse. Her knowledge of **story grammar** was also somewhat impaired. The woman with Covid-19 infection in case study 9 was under-informative in most discourse production tasks and had poor **letter fluency** performance. While none of these discourse anomalies can be directly linked to **executive dysfunction**, and there are many adults *without* neurodegenerative disorders who also omit and repeat information in narrative discourse, the consistent pattern of discourse impairment across several neurodegenerative disorders is strongly suggestive of a role for executive dysfunction in the language impairments of these adults.

The case studies also examined another cognitive ability that is known to deteriorate in neurodegeneration. That ability is **theory of mind** (ToM) or **social cognition**. ToM is the ability to attribute cognitive and **affective mental states** both to one's own mind and to the minds of others. ToM allows us to predict and explain the behaviour of others. The literature is replete with studies and reviews that demonstrate that people with neurodegeneration have impaired cognitive and affective ToM.[12–15] The functional consequences of ToM impairments are particularly evident at the pragmatic and discourse levels of language. People with neurodegeneration and ToM impairment may fail to attribute **communicative intentions** to speakers, leading to problems of **utterance interpretation**. A hearer may fail to recover the sarcastic intent with which an utterance is expressed, for example. ToM impairment may also result in a failure to attribute mental states to characters in a scene or in a story, or in the attribution of the wrong mental states to protagonists. More generally, there may be a reduction of language that expresses cognitive mental states (e.g. *knowledge, beliefs*) and affective mental states (e.g. *anger, happiness*) and a predominance of action-oriented language. These ToM difficulties were evident in several of the adults featured in the case studies.

In the Cookie Theft picture description task, few adults with neurodegeneration captured the mental states of the mother in the scene – she had *forgotten* to turn off the tap because she was *daydreaming*. In fact, the man with MND in case study 7 explicitly remarked that he did not know why the mother had not noticed that the water was overflowing. Similarly, none of the participants mentioned that the young girl was gesturing to her brother to be quiet because she *wanted* the theft of the cookies to pass undetected. During the Flowerpot Incident, the gentleman who was struck on the head by a flowerpot was *angry* and entered the building because he *wanted* to remonstrate with the owner of the apartment. Also, the woman gave the gentleman's dog a bone because she *wanted* to make amends for the injury that her falling flowerpot had caused. The man with LBD in case study 4 neglected to mention any of these mental states, with the result that the actions of the protagonists in his story appeared to lack motivation and purpose. Other participants misunderstood the intentions of the gentleman who kissed the elderly woman on the hand. He *wanted* to thank the woman for her **gesture** of kindness towards his dog, not invite her out for a date, as remarked by the adult with ARBD in case study 8. These difficulties in using mental state language, either appropriately or not at all, suggest that impaired ToM may also be contributing to the language problems of these adults with neurodegeneration.

Are Language Impairments Present in Adults with Neurodegeneration Without Dementia or Cognitive Impairment?

None of the participants in these case studies had been diagnosed with **dementia**. Moreover, their interaction and performance during home visits by the author and online meetings clearly indicated that they were not experiencing dementia. Each participant was alert, well oriented to time, space and person, and displayed behaviours appropriate to context. So, where language impairments arose in these individuals, they did so in the absence of dementia. To the extent that almost all participants had diagnosed or self-reported cognitive difficulties, it was more difficult to conclude that language impairments also occurred in adults with neurodegeneration without cognitive impairment. However, the findings of studies suggest that this may indeed be the case. PD individuals with normal cognitive status have been found to have difficulties in providing definitions and in sentence construction. Those with below normal cognitive status additionally display deficits in naming, interpreting ambiguous and **figurative**

language and semantic verbal fluency.[16] Grammatical and morphological impairments have been reported in individuals with genetically confirmed HD who are pre-symptomatic (i.e. not yet displaying symptoms, including cognitive impairments).[17,18] Further research is needed to establish if language impairment is actually coincident with normal cognitive status in individuals with neurodegeneration, or if subtle cognitive deficits are present but are undetectable using current assessment tools.

Are Adults with Neurodegeneration Adept at Compensating for Their Speech and Language Impairments?

Compensation for speech and language impairments may be achieved through several means. For an individual with **word-finding difficulty**, the use of manual gestures, pointing and mime may take the place of a word that the speaker cannot produce. A hearer can effectively compensate for his or her impaired comprehension of language by drawing on features of context and using knowledge of how events typically unfold in the world. Background knowledge tells a hearer who cannot decode the passive construction in the utterance '*The mouse was chased by the cat*' that it is the cat who did the chasing. This is because we expect cats to chase mice based on our knowledge of the world. A speaker can avoid the use of words or syntactic constructions that may prove difficult to produce by talking around a target word (**circumlocution**) and reformulating an utterance. Use of an augmentative or alternative communication (AAC) system also provides effective compensation for impaired speech and language. Conversational partners may also serve to compensate for a speaker's communication difficulties, although we will address this type of compensation subsequently.

The use of compensatory strategies by the adults with neurodegeneration in these case studies was quite limited. For the most part, this was because participants were reasonably competent verbal communicators even without the use of compensatory strategies. But other factors also played a role. The woman with HD and the man with MND in case studies 3 and 7, respectively, were unable to use manual gestures to support communication because of their severe motor disabilities. The man with **Parkinson's disease** in case study 6 tended to run out of expiratory air for speech before he completed his utterances. He actively compensated for this speech production difficulty by shortening his linguistic utterances. **Pronouns** like '*I*' that could be assumed in context were omitted from utterances wherever possible (e.g. "used to do grant work"), with the result that he was able to complete utterances without running out of breath. The participant with CBD in case study 1 displayed some problems with auditory verbal comprehension. However, he appeared able to use key words in questions (e.g. *hobbies, retirement*) to activate his background knowledge and to structure relevant, appropriate responses. This participant also used circumlocution when he was unable to retrieve target words. Finally, none of the participants used an AAC system to support their communication, a sign of their relative competence as verbal communicators.

Do Impaired and Preserved Language Skills Co-exist, Even Within the Same Level of Language?

There were numerous instances in these case studies where impaired and preserved language skills co-exist at the same language level. In terms of **syntax**, the woman with HD in case study 3 was able to use a range of **clauses**, **passive voice** constructions and **topicalisation**. However, she also abandoned many grammatical constructions. Having started these constructions, she did not appear to know how to complete them. In terms of **lexical semantics**, the man with CBD in case study 1 made many errors during **confrontation naming**. Notwithstanding his difficulty with **lexical retrieval**, this participant actively contributed to the author's **cueing** strategies. This suggested he retained considerable lexical-semantic knowledge of the target words even as he could not retrieve them from his mental lexicon. Preserved and impaired skills were also observed at the level of **pragmatics**. The man with PSP in case study 2 displayed a tendency for literal interpretation alongside an ability to use **deixis** and **presupposition** and engage in **conversational repair**. In terms of **discourse**, the adult with ARBD in case study 8 made effective use of **cohesion** but had difficulty drawing temporal-causal **inferences**. We can draw an important lesson from these patterns. **Speech-language pathologists** typically focus on deficits, a tendency that has resulted in the neglect of residual language skills that an individual with neurodegeneration can still use. This has had the unfortunate consequence of leading clinicians to overlook language skills that may be usefully leveraged in intervention.

Do Adults with Neurodegenerative Disorders Exhibit Impairments of Linguistic Competence, Communicative Competence, or Both?

The concept of **linguistic competence** is taken to represent our innate knowledge of the **grammar** of our language. As defined by **Chomsky**, grammar subsumes phonology, syntax and semantics. These levels of language contribute linguistic structures to the utterances we use. Adults with neurodegeneration can have marked impairments of linguistic structure (e.g. in progressive **aphasias**) that cause them to communicate inadequately. But it is also possible for adults with neurodegeneration to have impaired communication skills that cannot be accounted for by impairments of linguistic structure. In such a case, it is helpful to conceive of a separate concept of **communicative competence**. Communicative competence goes beyond knowledge of the structures of language to include judgements about what is being communicated and how it is being communicated. These judgements are associated with the pragmatic and discourse levels of language. They guide the contributions we make to conversation and our ability to narrate a story, describe a scene and convey instructions to others. There are many adults with neurodegeneration who have impairments of communicative competence even as their linguistic competence is relatively intact. They communicate more poorly than their linguistic skills would predict. Other adults with neurodegeneration can compensate for impaired linguistic competence and go on to communicate effectively. Still others have impairments of both types of competence.

Concepts of linguistic and communicative competence can be usefully applied to the case-study participants. The participant with CBD in case study 1 displayed phonological and grammatical errors and had poor **confrontation naming** and **word-finding difficulty** in conversation. His linguistic competence was clearly compromised. Yet, he retained considerable strengths in conversation and **discourse**. He was able to contribute relevant, informative utterances to conversation, used idiomatic language appropriately and corrected misunderstandings. He was also able to use **cohesion** in discourse and retained knowledge of narrative structure. Such difficulties as existed in **pragmatics** and discourse – erroneous **inferences** and the omission, repetition and incorrect sequencing of information – were not so clearly related to impaired linguistic structure and suggested an independent contribution from cognition to communicative competence. Other case-study participants had intact linguistic competence and yet still had communication difficulties. The woman with MS in case study 5 displayed intact phonology, syntax and semantics. However, she exhibited several discourse deficits. She often drew mistaken inferences in discourse, leading to a misinterpretation of events. She omitted information from narratives and had impaired knowledge of **story grammar**. None of these weaknesses in her communicative competence were predicted by her linguistic competence which was intact. This same profile of impairment was evident in the man with ARBD in case study 8 who had problems drawing inferences in discourse alongside intact linguistic competence.

Do Conversational Partners Facilitate or Dominate Exchanges with Adults Who Have Neurodegenerative Disorders?

Neurodegeneration typically emerges in later life when patients and their spouses have already established a certain style or pattern of communication. In some communication dyads, one partner is more dominant than the other and assumes control of the conversational exchange. Other communication dyads are more collaborative in nature, with each partner making an equal contribution to the development of a conversation. With the emergence of illness such as neurodegeneration, these pre-existing styles of communication can often assume a more exaggerated form. This was evident in some of the patient–spouse dyads in these case studies. The spouse of the man with PSP in case study 2 adopted a highly directive communication style. It included the asking of questions to which the spouse knew the answers (e.g. *What countries did we pass through?*), the use of explicit commands (e.g. *Tell Louise about the library*), sound and syllable cues (e.g. *mu, mu, Germany, Munich*), letter cues (e.g. *begins with an R*), sentence completion (e.g. *From there you went to...*), and explicit corrections (e.g. *No, you went to Queens first*). This communication style had the effect of limiting her partner's contributions to conversation and reducing his role to that of a passive respondent. In some neurodegenerative dyads, this may lead to patient stress and frustration and reduced quality of life.[19] It was not possible to establish if this was the case for the individual with PSP in case study 2 who displayed no overt frustration at the high level of direction adopted by his spouse.

A more collaborative style of communication was also evident in the patient–spouse dyads in the case studies. The man with CBD in case study 1 had **word-finding difficulty** in conversation. Rather than adopt an unnatural **cueing** strategy like the spouse described above, his wife waited to be invited to produce the target word, as the following exchange illustrates:

PAR: we had to do two, what would you call it?
SPO: talks

In case study 6, the man with PD encouraged participation from his spouse when he was trying to recall how long it had been since he was last out on his boat. Of equal interest is the way in which his spouse corrected his response. Instead of saying '*No, it was three years*', as the spouse of the man with PSP did, the partner in this case avoided explicitly correcting her husband by acknowledging his response and then revising it:

INV: when were you last out on the boat?
PAR: few year ago now, wasn't it (.) two years
SPO: be over two, three years nearly

In case study 7, the man with MND and his wife jointly constructed part of his response to a question about holidays that he had undertaken. Rather than issue a command like *Tell Louise about your trip to Tuscany*, as the spouse of the man with PSP did, a statement was produced which the man with MND could choose to develop as he pleased:

INV: do you have a holiday that you've had that you've really enjoyed very positive memories about?
...

PAR: we've had a few
SPO: your fiftieth birthday one to Italy to Tuscany

PAR: that was a pretty enjoyable one when we went to Tuscany for a fortnight with friends

In each of these examples, a more collaborative style of communication is adopted in the patient–spouse dyad. This less directive style of communication makes more opportunities for communication available to people with **neuro-degenerative disorders** and is associated with higher ratings of patient satisfaction with the communication event.[20]

References

[1] Boschi, V., Catricalà, E., Consonni, M., Chesi, C., Moro, A. and Cappa, S.F. (2017) 'Connected speech in neurodegenerative language disorders: A review', *Frontiers in Psychology*, 8: 269. doi: 10.3389/fpsyg.2017.00269.

[2] Peterson, K.A., Patterson, K. and Rowe, J.B. (2019) 'Language impairment in progressive supranuclear palsy and corticobasal syndrome', *Journal of Neurology*, doi:10.1007/s00415-019-09463-1.

[3] Catricalà, E., Boschi, V., Cuoco, S., Galiano, F., Picillo, M., Gobbi, E., Miozzo, A., Chesi, C., Esposito, V., Santangelo, G., Pellecchia, M.T., Borsa, V.M., Barone, P., Garrard, P., Iannaccone, S. and Cappa, S.F. (2019) 'The language profile of progressive supranuclear palsy', *Cortex*, 115: 294–308.

[4] Daniele, A., Barbier, A., Di Giuda, D., Vita, M.G., Piccininni, C., Spinelli, P., Tondo, G., Fasano, A., Colosimo, C., Giordano, A. and Gainotti, G. (2013) 'Selective impairment of action-verb naming and comprehension in progressive supranuclear palsy', *Cortex*, 49 (4): 948–960.

[5] Gagnon, M., Barrette, J. and Macoir, J. (2018) 'Language disorders in Huntington disease: A systematic literature review', *Cognitive and Behavioral Neurology*, 31 (4): 179–192.

[6] Chenery, H.J., Copland, D.A. and Murdoch, B.E. (2010) 'Complex language functions and subcortical mechanisms: Evidence from Huntington's disease and patients with non-thalamic subcortical lesions', *International Journal of Language & Communication Disorders*, 37 (4): 459–474.

[7] Jensen, A.M., Chenery, H.J. and Copland, D.A. (2006) 'A comparison of picture description abilities in individuals with vascular subcortical lesions and Huntington's disease', *Journal of Communication Disorders*, 39 (1): 62–77.

[8] Bayles, K., McCullough, K. and Tomoeda, C. (2020) *Cognitive-Communication Disorders of MCI and Dementia: Definition, Assessment, and Clinical Management*, Third Edition. San Diego, CA: Plural Publishing.

[9] Gross, R.G., Ash, S., McMillan, C.T., Gunawardena, D., Powers, C., Libon, D.J., Moore, P., Liang, T.W. and Grossman, M. (2010) 'Impaired information integration contributes to communication difficulty in corticobasal syndrome', *Cognitive and Behavioral Neurology*, 23 (1): 1–7.

[10] Ellis, C., Crosson, B., Gonzalez Rothi, L.J., Okun, M.S. and Rosenbek, J.C. (2015) 'Narrative discourse cohesion in early stage Parkinson's disease', *Journal of Parkinson's Disease*, 5 (2): 403–411.

[11] Ash, S., McMillan, C., Gross, R.G., Cook, P., Morgan, B., Boiler, A., Dreyfuss, M., Siderowf, A. and Grossman, M. (2011) 'The organization of narrative discourse in Lewy body spectrum disorder', *Brain and Language*, 119 (1): 30–41.

[12] Cummings, L. (2020) *Language in Dementia*. Cambridge: Cambridge University Press.

[13] Cummings, L. (2009) *Clinical Pragmatics*. Cambridge: Cambridge University Press.

[14] Cummings, L. (2014) 'Pragmatic disorders and theory of mind', in L. Cummings (ed.) *Cambridge Handbook of Communication Disorders*. Cambridge: Cambridge University Press, 559–577.

[15] Cummings, L. (2013) 'Clinical pragmatics and theory of mind', in A. Capone, F. Lo Piparo & M. Carapezza (eds), *Perspectives on Linguistic Pragmatics*, Series: Perspectives in Pragmatics, Philosophy & Psychology, Vol. 2. Cham, Switzerland: Springer International Publishing AG, 23–56.

[16] Lewis, F.M., Lapointe, L.L., Murdoch, B.E. and Chenery, H.J. (1998) 'Language impairment in Parkinson's disease', *Aphasiology*, 12 (3): 193–206.

[17] Németh, D., Dye, C.D., Sefcsik, T., Janacsek, K., Turi, Z., Londe, Z., Klivenyi, P., Kincses, T., Nikoletta, S., Vecsei, L. and Ullman, M.T. (2012) 'Language deficits in pre-symptomatic Huntington's disease: Evidence from Hungarian', *Brain and Language*, 121 (3): 248–253.

[18] Hinzen, W., Rosselló, J., Morey, C., Camara, E., Garcia-Gorro, C., Salvador, R. and de Diego-Balaguer, R. (2018) 'A systematic linguistic profile of spontaneous narrative speech in pre-symptomatic and early stage Huntington's disease', *Cortex*, 100: 71–83.

[19] Downs, M. and Collins, L. (2015) 'Person-centred communication in dementia care', *Nursing Standard*, 30 (11): 37–41.

[20] Kindell, J., Keady, J., Sage, K. and Wilkinson, R. (2017) 'Everyday conversation in dementia: A review of the literature to inform research and practice', *International Journal of Language & Communication Disorders*, 52 (4): 392–406.

GLOSSARY

Adductor jerk Tapping the patellar tendon can sometimes elicit not only a knee jerk on that side but also a crossed thigh adductor jerk. This should be considered a normal finding in the first months of life. Later, however, brisk and crossed thigh adductor jerks are associated with upper motor neuron damage.

Adverb An open word class that can modify adjectives (e.g. very pretty), adverbs (e.g. rather quickly) and verbs (walked quickly). Many adverbs are formed by adding the suffix −ly to an adjective (e.g. loud → loudly). However, there are many adverbs in English where this pattern does not apply (e.g. soon, very).

Aetiology The medical or other causes of a disorder. Dementia may have genetic, infectious, metabolic, vascular or iatrogenic factors in its aetiology.

Affective mental state A mental state the content of which is an emotion like happiness, fear or disgust. Affective mental states may be established through the processing of facial expressions and linguistic utterances (e.g. I am really unhappy today). An ability to attribute affective mental states to another person's mind is called affective theory of mind.

Agent see semantic role

Akinesia This refers to a poverty of spontaneous movement (e.g. in facial expression) or associated movement (e.g. arm swinging during walking). Freezing and prolonged time to initiate movement are other manifestations of akinesia. Akinesia is a feature of Parkinson's disease where it is often used synonymously with the term 'bradykinesia'.

Alcohol-related brain damage An umbrella term that covers the various psychoneurological/cognitive conditions associated with long-term alcohol misuse and related vitamin deficiencies. The term includes Wernicke-Korsakoff syndrome at the more extreme end as well as less severe frontal lobe dysfunctions.

Alzheimer's disease The most common form of dementia, accounting for 60% to 80% of all dementia cases. Alzheimer's dementia is characterised by prominent episodic memory impairment, with secondary deficits in word-finding skills, spatial cognition and executive functions.

Amygdala A group of nuclei located in the anterior medial portion of the brain's temporal lobe. The amygdala is part of the limbic system. It is involved in processing emotions, particularly fear, although its constituent nuclei have diverse functions.

Amyotrophic lateral sclerosis see *motor neuron disease*

Anaphoric reference A form of cohesion in which there is reference to a preceding textual unit (known as the antedecent). In the following example, the pronoun *it* in the second sentence refers to the noun phrase *a red dress* in the first sentence: Mary bought a red dress. It was very expensive.

Anomia A word-finding difficulty in which a client is unable to evoke, retrieve or recall a particular word. In anomic aphasia, there are relatively severe word-finding problems in the context of fluent, grammatically well-formed speech production and relatively intact auditory comprehension.

Anomic aphasia see *anomia*

Anxiety An emotion which is characterised by feelings of tension, worried thoughts and physical symptoms such as increased blood pressure. Anxiety is a neuropsychiatric symptom of many forms of dementia.

Apathy A clinically significant loss of motivation or lack of interest. Apathy is a psychological symptom of all forms of dementia.

Aphasia An acquired language disorder in which the expression and/or reception of language (spoken, written and signed) is compromised. Aphasia can be broadly classified as fluent and non-fluent types. Fluent aphasia is further subdivided into Wernicke's, anomic, conduction and transcortical sensory aphasia. Non-fluent aphasia is further subdivided into Broca's and transcortical motor aphasia. A further non-fluent aphasia – global aphasia – is characterised by severe impairment of all language functions.

Apomorphine A dopamine agonist drug that acts like dopamine and is used to control the symptoms of Parkinson's disease. Apomorphine is administered by injection or continuous infusion using a pump.

Apraxia A motor disorder which can affect speech production (apraxia of speech), the movement of limbs (limb apraxia) and the movement of oral structures (oral apraxia). Adults with dementia can experience one or more of these forms of apraxia. For example, limb apraxia is often found in clients with vascular dementia while apraxia of speech can occur in clients with primary progressive aphasia.

Apraxia of speech A motor programming disorder which has its onset in adulthood typically following a stroke. Speech intelligibility is reduced in the absence of neuromuscular weakness. As well as speech errors involving consonants and vowels, AOS speakers display inconsistent errors, have more difficulty with volitional speech production than automatic speech production, and can display articulatory groping. Apraxia of speech may occur in isolation or alongside oral apraxia.

Argument structure The lexical representation of argument-taking lexical items such as verbs and prepositions. The argument structure indicates the number of arguments a lexical item takes (e.g. three arguments in the preposition '*x* is between *y* and *z*'), the syntactic expression of the arguments and their semantic relation to the lexical item.

Arrhythmia This is a problem with the rate or rhythm of the heartbeat. During an arrhythmia, the heart can beat too fast (tachycardia), too slowly (bradycardia) or with an irregular rhythm.

Articulation The production of speech sounds through the coordinated action of articulators such as the lips, tongue, jaw and velum. Articulation is impaired in motor speech disorders like dysarthria and apraxia of speech.

Ataxia Impaired coordination of voluntary muscle movement that is usually caused by cerebellar dysfunction or impaired vestibular or proprioceptive afferent input to the cerebellum. Ataxia can have many different aetiologies including cerebellar haemorrhage and neurodegenerative disease.

Atrophy When applied to the brain, atrophy is the loss of brain tissue due to neurodegeneration (e.g. Alzheimer's disease), cranial irradiation, vascular factors and ageing.

Attention A state of focused awareness on a subset of the perceptual information available in the environment. Attention is an executive function which is mediated by the frontostriatal circuit in the brain. There are different types of attention. For example, selective attention is the differential processing of multiple sources of information that are available simultaneously.

Augmentative and alternative communication When spoken communication skills are impaired and are likely to deteriorate further, as in neurodegeneration, a type of AAC may be considered for use with a client. AAC may take high- and low-tech forms such as a communication board attached to a client's wheelchair or the use of synthesized speech output.

Autoimmune disorder A disorder in which the body's own immune system produces antibodies that attack its tissues. Autoimmune diseases include neurological disorders such as Guillain-Barré syndrome, multiple sclerosis and myasthenia gravis.

Autonomic disorder Any disorder of the autonomic nervous system which controls cardiovascular and respiratory function, body temperature, gastrointestinal motility, urinary and sexual function, and metabolic and endocrine physiology.

Axial rigidity see *progressive supranuclear palsy*

Bradykinesia The slowness of a performed movement, and one of the cardinal motor symptoms of Parkinson's disease. Bradykinesia is often used interchangeably with hypokinesia and akinesia, although these terms mean different things. While bradykinesia describes decreased velocity of movement, hypokinesia refers to the decreased amplitude of movement, and akinesia is an inability or difficulty initiating movement.

Bulbar symptom Dysarthria, dysphagia, sialorrhoea (drooling), aspiration and pseudobulbar affect (laughter or crying that is not consistent with mood) are bulbar symptoms. These symptoms are associated with pathology of the following cranial nerves: glossopharyngeal (IX); vagus (X); accessory (XI); and hypoglossal (XII). The causes of bulbar pathology are vascular (infarction of the medulla), neurodegenerative (motor neuron disease), neoplastic (brainstem tumour), inflammatory (poliomyelitis) and genetic in nature.

Category fluency see *verbal fluency*

Caudate nucleus The caudate nucleus is anatomically associated with the lateral ventricle and follows its curvature. Its head is located within the frontal lobe, its body is located in the parietal lobe, and its tail goes into the temporal lobe. The caudate and putamen collectively comprise the neostriatum. Atrophy of the caudate nucleus occurs in Huntington's disease.

Central nervous system The part of the nervous system that consists of the brain and spinal cord.

Cerebellar sign Diseases of the cerebellum lead to clinical signs that occur throughout the body. Three such signs are scanning speech, nystagmus and acute cerebellar ataxia (a wide-based and staggering gait).

Cerebrospinal fluid A fluid that is produced by the choroid plexuses in the ventricles of the brain. Cerebrospinal fluid is found in the subarachnoid space between two of the meninges (pia mater and arachnoid) that protect the brain and spinal cord.

Cholecystectomy Surgical removal of the gall bladder.

Chomsky, Noam An American academic, born in 1928, who is best known for his contribution to linguistics but also for his political views. Chomsky argued that knowledge of language (so-called linguistic competence) is an innate biological capacity of humans that children bring to the learning of their native language. Chomsky has been a faculty member of the Massachusetts Institute of Technology (MIT) since 1955.

Chorea Involuntary, irregular, arrhythmic, non-patterned, purposeless movements that flow randomly from one body part to another. Huntington's disease is the most common cause of inherited chorea. Chorea can also be found in acquired disorders that have infectious (e.g. HIV), immune-mediated (e.g. systemic lupus erythematosus) or metabolic (e.g. renal failure) causes.

Chronic fatigue syndrome Also known as myalgic encephalomyelitis, chronic fatigue syndrome is a complex, chronic medical condition that is characterised by symptom clusters. Symptoms include pathological fatigue and malaise which worsens with exertion, immune and cognitive dysfunction, unrefreshing sleep, pain, neuroendocrine and immune symptoms, and autonomic dysfunction.

Circumlocution   The literal meaning of this word is to talk ('locution') around ('circum') a word. Circumlocutions are used by aphasic speakers and speakers with dementia when they cannot retrieve a target word. A speaker with primary progressive aphasia (PPA) who says 'a good witch' for *fairy godmother* is using circumlocution.

Cirrhosis   The pathological end-stage of any chronic liver disease. Cirrhosis most commonly results from chronic hepatitis B and C, alcohol-related liver disease and non-alcoholic fatty liver disease.

Clause   A clause consists of a main or lexical verb, any elements required by the main verb (e.g. subject) and any optional elements that a speaker or writer may decide to include. When a clause is not part of a larger clause, it is known as a main clause or sentence.

Clonus   A rhythmic, oscillating stretch reflex that is related to lesions in the upper motor neurons and is generally accompanied by hyperreflexia. It is part of a neurological examination. An example of clonus is when a clinician taps the patellar tendon once lightly and a series of obvious repeated knee extensions and relaxations continues for a dozen beats.

Cogwheeling   This describes the regular ratchet-like quality to resistance that occurs when the limb of a patient with Parkinson's disease is moved passively.

Cohesion   see *cohesive device*

Cohesive device   Certain grammatical and lexical features of sentences can link them to other sentences of a text. Forms of cohesion include anaphoric reference (e.g. Paul *likes marathons.* He *completes one every year*), substitution (e.g. *Jane bought* an expensive sofa. *It was the* one *in the shop window*), lexical reiteration (e.g. *The* man *and woman left the party early. The* man *was tired*), and ellipsis (e.g. *Would anyone like a drink? I would*).

Communication disorder   Any impairment of verbal and non-verbal communication. Communication disorders include speech, language, hearing, fluency and voice disorders. They are assessed and treated by speech-language pathologists.

Communicative competence   The body of knowledge that enables speakers and hearers to make use of, and interpret, linguistic utterances and non-verbal behaviours (e.g. gesture) in a communicative exchange. Communicative competence involves complex judgements about how utterances are used in context. A speaker can have intact linguistic competence, and still communicate inadequately because of compromised communicative competence.

Communicative intention   A mental state that has significance in utterance interpretation. A hearer cannot be said to have understood a speaker's utterance unless they are able to establish the communicative intention which motivated the speaker to produce it.

Compensatory strategy   Any type of behavioural adjustment, either explicitly taught or naturally acquired, that compensates for a deficit in communication. For example, an adult with Parkinson's disease may reduce the length of spoken utterances by omitting redundant language to compensate for reduced breath support for speech.

Computerised axial tomography (CAT or CT scan) A technique in which an X-ray source produces a narrow, fan-shaped beam of X-rays to irradiate a section of the body. On a single rotation of the X-ray source around the body, many different 'snapshots' are taken. These are then reconstructed by a computer into a cross-sectional image of internal organs and tissues for each complete rotation.

Confrontation naming The presentation of an object or picture of an object which a subject is required to name. Confrontation naming is used to assess lexical retrieval.

Conjunctivitis Inflammation of the conjunctiva, the protective membrane that lines the inner eyelids and covers the outer surface of the eyeballs. There are different forms of conjunctivitis (e.g. allergic, infectious). The most common form, acute infectious conjunctivitis, is mostly caused by bacteria and viruses.

Content word Words that convey most meaning in a sentence. Content words belong to open classes like noun (e.g. *table, holiday*), verb (e.g. *play, run*), adjective (e.g. *tasty, solid*) and adverb (e.g. *fast, hastily*).

Convergence impairment A common vision disorder in which a person's eyes tend to drift outwards when they try to use their eyes together up close. Once an object is brought to within 10 cm of the bridge of their nose, affected patients are unable to converge.

Conversational dyad The two-person structure that is the basis of all communication. In a clinical context, dyads can include any of the following conversational participants: patient–therapist; caregiver–patient; and spouse–patient.

Conversational repair Trouble sources can arise during conversation and need to be repaired by participants. Repair work can be initiated either by the speaker who is responsible for a trouble source (self-initiated repair) or by the hearer (other-initiated repair). The speaker who utters *I want a new dress, um hat for the wedding*, undertakes a self-initiated repair that is unprompted by the hearer. Repair work is often achieved collaboratively, especially in clients with neurodegenerative disorders.

Coordination The conjoining of two or more elements of equal syntactic status using the coordinating conjunctions *and, or* and *but*. The elements so conjoined may be nouns (e.g. *John likes wine* and *cheese*), adjectives (e.g. *The dog is wet* and *dirty*), adverbs (e.g. *They worked quickly* and *competently*), or clauses (e.g. *Fran likes Spain* but *Paul likes France*).

Corticobasal degeneration A neurodegenerative disease that is caused by the accumulation of hyperphosphorylated four-repeat tau isoforms. The disease is characterised by asymmetric cortical dysfunction that often affects motor control of a limb, along with executive dysfunction, rigidity, a jerky postural tremor, myoclonus, dystonia and a gait disorder. Speech may be compromised as a result of apraxia and non-fluent aphasia.

Cranial nerve   Twelve paired sets of nerves that arise from the brain or brain-stem and leave the central nervous system through cranial foraminae. These nerves control motor and sensory functions of the head and neck. Several cranial nerves are important for speech, hearing and swallowing.

Cueing   The delivery of a verbal or non-verbal prompt to elicit a response (usually a target word) from a client. In order to elicit the target word 'watch' from an adult with aphasia, for example, a speech-language pathologist may produce the initial sound of the word (phonemic cue), may say 'This is the thing you use to tell the time' (semantic cue), or may gesture looking at a watch on her wrist (gestural cue).

Deictic expression   (or deixis) Linguistic expressions can be used to 'point' to aspects of spatiotemporal, social and discourse context. There are five types of deixis: personal (*I want to leave early*), social (*Wie heißen Sie?*), temporal (*Sally departed last week*), spatial (*Joe lives here*) and discourse deixis (*The next section will present a different view*).

Deixis   see *deictic expression*

Delirium   A common and serious acute neuropsychiatric syndrome with core features of inattention and global cognitive dysfunction. The aetiologies of delirium are diverse and multifactorial and include acute medical illness, medical complication or drug intoxication. One of the most prominent risk factors for delirium among elderly patients is dementia.

Delusion   A false and bizarre belief. Delusions are a positive symptom of schizophrenia and a neuropsychiatric symptom of dementia.

Dementia   Deterioration of higher cortical functions (e.g. language, memory) that can be caused by a range of diseases (e.g. vascular disease, Alzheimer's disease), infections (e.g. HIV infection) and lifestyle (e.g. alcohol-related dementia).

Demonstrative pronoun   The words *this/that* and *these/those* can also stand alone as pronouns in a sentence, e.g. This *is tastier than* that. Some uses of demonstrative pronouns refer to non-linguistic context (e.g. This *is bright red* where *this* may refer to a dress). Other uses can refer to preceding text (e.g. That *was a clear explanation*) and are known as anaphoric pronouns.

Demyelination   A pathological process that describes the loss of myelin from nerve cells with relative preservation of axons. This process occurs in diseases such as multiple sclerosis that damage myelin sheaths or the cells that form them. Demyelinated axons tend to atrophy and may eventually degenerate.

Depression   A common mental disorder that is characterised by sadness, loss of interest or pleasure, feelings of guilt or low self-worth, disturbed sleep or appetite, feelings of tiredness and poor concentration.

Derivational morphology   A type of morphemic word formation which includes prefixation and suffixation. Whereas inflectional morphemes generate word forms (e.g. *walks, walking, walked*), derivational morphemes generate new words (e.g. *discover, discovery, discoverable*).

Derivational suffix   see *suffix*

Dialect   The pronunciation, lexemes, grammatical structures and discourse features of a particular variety of a language.

Diplopia   Diplopia or double vision may be monocular or binocular. Monocular diplopia is usually the result of ocular abnormalities such as a dislocated lens, although it may also result from psychogenic factors. Binocular diplopia results from misalignment of both eyes. It is the form of diplopia that is most characteristic of a neurological disorder.

Direct reported speech   In direct reported speech, the reporting speaker presents the reported speaker's words in the form of a direct quotation (e.g. *Joan said "That meal was cold and too salty"*). In indirect reported speech, the reported speaker's words are presented in the form of a paraphrase (e.g. *Joan said that the meal was cold and too salty*).

Discourse   In terms of linguistic analysis, discourse is the level of language above individual sentences. The focus of study is on extended extracts of language in spoken and written texts.

Dopamine   A neurotransmitter that is involved in the regulation of a variety of functions, including locomotor activity, emotion and affect, and neuroendocrine secretion. Dopaminergic neurons in the substantia nigra pars compacta are the main source of dopamine in the central nervous system. The loss of these neurons is associated with Parkinson's disease.

Drooling   Also known as sialorrhea or ptyalis, drooling occurs when there is excess saliva in the mouth beyond the lip margin. Parkinson's disease is the most common cause of drooling in adults where it is associated with reduced swallowing and not excessive saliva production. Drooling can have an adverse impact on social functioning, and can result in aspiration, skin deterioration, bad odour and infections.

Duopa   A form of carbidopa/levodopa that is used to treat the motor symptoms of Parkinson's disease. A pump delivers Duopa directly into the small intestine via a tube. This improves absorption of the drug and reduces 'off' times when the drug is no longer working and symptoms such as tremor re-emerge.

Dysarthria   A speech disorder that is caused by damage to the central and peripheral nervous systems. Dysarthria can be developmental or acquired in nature and affects articulation, resonation, respiration, phonation and prosody.

Dysphagia   The term given to a swallowing disorder in children and adults. Dysphagia can arise following a stroke or other neurological injury (neurogenic dysphagia), as a result of structural causes (e.g. a tumour), as a complication of surgery (iatrogenic dysphagia) or on account of psychological factors (psychogenic dysphagia). The oral and pharyngeal stages of swallowing may be compromised (oropharyngeal dysphagia) or the impairment may occur in the oesophageal stage of swallowing (oesophageal dysphagia). In most cases, the disorder can be managed by dietary and other modifications. When dysphagia is severe, non-oral feeding is instituted as the only safe method of feeding.

Dysphoria   A low mood that may include chronic dissatisfaction, restlessness or depression.

Dystonia   A movement disorder in which there is twisting, involuntary contractions of antagonistic muscles that cause repetitive movements or abnormal posture. Dystonia may occur in isolation or in combination with other movement disorders and is a feature of neurodegenerative diseases such as Huntington's disease.

Ellipsis   A form of grammatical cohesion in which there is omission of elements that are required by grammatical rules. For example, the question *Who would like beans on toast?* may receive the elliptical response *I would*.

Epidemiology   The study of the distribution of diseases and disorders in populations. Epidemiologists investigate the prevalence (total number of cases in a population) and incidence (number of newly diagnosed cases, typically within a year) of disorders in populations. They also investigate the distribution of diseases according to factors such as gender, age, socioeconomic class and ethnicity.

Epstein–Barr virus   Also known as human herpes virus 4, the Epstein-Barr virus (EBV) is a member of the herpes virus family. It is spread most commonly through bodily fluids, mostly saliva, and can cause infectious mononucleosis (glandular fever) and other illnesses. There is no vaccine to protect against EBV infection. Antibodies showing current or past EBV infection can be found in about nine out of ten adults.

Euthymia   A transdiagnostic concept that refers to the presence of positive affects and psychological well-being.

Executive dysfunction   Executive functions are a group of cognitive skills which are essential to goal-directed behaviour (e.g. planning ability, mental flexibility) and which are believed to be mediated in large part by the brain's frontal lobes. Impairment of these cognitive skills results in executive dysfunction which plays a role in cognitive-communication disorders in conditions like dementia and traumatic brain injury.

Executive function   see *executive dysfunction*

Fasciculation   Fine, rapid, flickering and sometimes worm-like twitching of a portion of muscle. In the tongue, fasciculations may be observed as small movements on the tongue surface. Fasciculations can be observed in healthy persons and in clients with neurological disorders (e.g. motor neuron disease).

Figurative language   Metaphorical, idiomatic and other non-literal language in which the meaning of an utterance is not derivable from the sum of its component words. Figurative language is not confined to literary texts but occurs in everyday language use.

Filler   Fillers are words and expressions such as *uh, um* and *like*. They have little or no semantic content, but still perform an important linguistic function. They allow speakers to retain the floor in conversation as they are planning how to produce an utterance.

Fine motor movement   The use of small motor muscles for tasks such as writing, buttoning and grasping objects.

Flail arm syndrome   An atypical presentation of ALS/MND that is characterised by progressive, predominantly proximal, weakness of upper limbs without involvement of the lower limb, bulbar or respiratory muscles. There is evidence that more men than women develop flail arm syndrome (the male: female ratio was 9:1 in one study[1]) and that patients with the syndrome have a prolonged survival compared to classical ALS/MND patients.[2]

Fluency   The production of speech in a rhythmic, smooth manner. Fluency is affected by aspects of speech production (e.g. good respiratory support for speech) and language (e.g. efficient lexical retrieval).

Gastroesophageal reflux disease   A gastrointestinal motility disorder that results from the reflux of stomach contents into the oesophagus or oral cavity resulting in symptoms or complications. The typical symptoms of GERD are heartburn and regurgitation of gastric contents into the oropharynx.

Gastroparesis   A digestive disorder in which the motility of the stomach is either abnormal or absent. In gastroparesis, the stomach is unable to contract normally, and therefore cannot crush or propel food into the small intestine properly.

Genetics   The branch of biology that deals with heredity, especially mechanisms of hereditary transmission, and variation of inherited characteristics among similar or related organisms.

Gesture   The use of the hands and other parts of the body for communicative purposes. Gesture may be used alongside speech or in place of speech during communication.

Grammar   The branch of linguistics that examines word structure (morphology) and sentence structure (syntax). For Chomsky, the grammar of language also contains phonological and semantic aspects.

Gross motor movement   The use of large muscle groups to coordinate the body movements needed to perform activities such as maintaining balance, walking, sitting upright, jumping and throwing objects.

Guillain-Barré syndrome   A rare, rapidly progressive condition in which there is inflammation of peripheral nerves (polyneuritis) causing muscle weakness and sometimes leading to complete paralysis. The disease is often preceded by a respiratory or gastrointestinal infection which produces an immune response that damages the axons or myelin sheaths of nerve cells. Miller-Fisher syndrome is a variant of Guillain-Barré syndrome that is characterised by abnormal muscle coordination with poor balance and clumsy walking, weakness or paralysis of the eye muscles, and absence of tendon reflexes.

Hallucination   The perception of things that do not exist. Hallucinations may be visual or auditory in nature. Hallucinations can occur in psychotic disorders like schizophrenia. They are also a neuropsychiatric symptom in dementia.

Hedging   A pragmatic device that allows a speaker to modify the definiteness of an utterance and the attitude of the speaker towards a proposition expressed by an utterance. Several linguistic features can perform hedging including modal auxiliary verbs (*She* might *attend the meeting*), probability adjectives (*It is* likely *that Mike will apply*), and phrases such as *I believe* and *to our knowledge* (*To our knowledge, the parcel was delivered on time*).

Humour   A technical expression which is intended to cover all pre-theoretical notions of comical, ridiculous or laughable language. Humour is a high-level language skill that is still being acquired into adolescence and young adulthood. Humour appreciation is often impaired early in dementia.

Huntington's disease   A neurodegenerative disease that is caused by a dominantly inherited Cytosine Adenine Guanine (CAG) trinucleotide repeat expansion in the huntingtin gene on chromosome 4. The main clinical features of the disease are movement disorder (principally, chorea and dystonia), cognitive impairments and neuropsychiatric problems.

Hyperbole   A type of figurative language that involves exaggeration, often for humorous effect, e.g. *She is older than the hills!*

Hypernasality   (also, hypernasal speech) Excessive nasal resonance in speech which may be caused by velopharyngeal incompetence. Hypernasality is a feature of dysarthric speech.

Hypertension   High blood pressure, defined as the average systolic blood pressure or diastolic blood pressure that is at or above 95th percentile for gender, age and height on three or more occasions. Hypertension is a major risk factor for mortality from cardiovascular diseases and the primary cause of stroke.

Hypokinetic dysarthria   A form of dysarthria that is associated with lesions of the basal ganglia and associated brainstem nuclei. Hypokinetic dysarthria is a feature of Parkinson's disease. All aspects of speech production may be compromised in Parkinson's disease, although disturbances of prosody, phonation and articulation are most common.

Hypometabolism   A common feature of many neurodegenerative diseases, hypometabolism is characterised by decreased brain glucose consumption.

Hypomimia   A cardinal sign of Parkinson's disease, hypomimia is characterised by a marked diminution of expressive gestures of the face, including brow movements that accompany speech and emotional facial expressions. Hypomimia is often present in only one side of the face.

Idiom   A linguistic expression the meaning of which cannot be based on the meanings of its individual words (i.e. the meaning of idiomatic expressions is non-compositional). Common idioms include *pop the question* and *let the cat out of the bag*. The understanding or comprehension of idioms is often compromised in clients with pragmatic disorders.

Idiopathic   Of unknown cause.

Impulsivity   Impulsivity is broadly defined as action without foresight. It is a feature of neurodegenerative disorders and psychiatric conditions, including attention deficit hyperactivity disorder, mania and substance abuse.

Incidence   The rate of occurrence of new cases of a disease or condition. Incidence is calculated by dividing the number of new cases of a disease or condition in a specified time period (usually a year) by the size of the population under consideration.

Inference   A cognitive process in which a conclusion is derived from premises. There are several different types of inferences which vary according to the strength of the warrant provided by the premises. Inferences are vital for pragmatic language understanding, although the exact nature of the inferences involved (deductive, inductive, etc.) is uncertain.

Infinitive clause   A subordinate clause that contains a *to*-infinitive, e.g. *Sally wants* <u>to leave early</u>. In this example, the *to*-infinitive clause functions as the object of the verb *wants*. However, *to*-infinitive clauses can also be the subject in a sentence, e.g. <u>To climb Mount Everest</u> *would be a truly amazing experience*.

Inflectional morphology   The branch of morphology which examines the use of bound inflectional morphemes like *–s, –ed* and *–ing* to generate word forms such as *walks, walked* and *walking*.

Inflectional suffix   see *suffix*

Inhibition   see *inhibitory control*

Inhibitory control   A central component of executive function, inhibitory control focuses on the ability to actively inhibit or delay a dominant response to achieve a goal. Inhibitory control is impaired in a wide range of neurodegenerative, neurological and psychiatric conditions including dementia, traumatic brain injury and schizophrenia.

Instrument   see *semantic role*

Intelligibility   The ease with which a hearer can understand the spoken output of a speaker. Speech disorders such as dysarthria and apraxia of speech can compromise a speaker's intelligibility. A highly unintelligible speaker may need to use an alternative communication system.

Intonation   The use of identifiable pitch patterns over stretches of speech to convey attitude and feelings (e.g. anger, surprise), grammatical categories (statements versus questions) and semantic content (completeness versus incompleteness).

Ischaemia   The insufficient supply of blood to an organ or tissue, usually as a result of blockage or narrowing of an artery. Tissue can be damaged if ischaemia is severe and there is an insufficient supply of oxygen and nutrients.

Keratoconus   A condition in which the normally round cornea becomes thin and develops a cone-like bulge.

Knee jerk reflex   Also known as the patellar tendon reflex, this reflex is tested by striking the patellar tendon inferior to the patella (kneecap) with a reflex hammer while the lower leg hangs freely off the edge of a bench. The knee jerk reflex is mediated by the L3 and L4 nerve roots, mainly L4. A normal or brisk knee jerk would have little more than one swing forward and one back.

Korsakoff's syndrome   A neuropsychiatric disorder associated with significant deficits in anterograde and retrograde memory. Immediate memory is maintained, but short-term memory is diminished with intact sensorium. Patients can fabricate stories in the setting of clear consciousness (confabulation). The disorder is caused by thiamine deficiency related to long-term alcohol abuse and arises when Wernicke's encephalopathy is left untreated, or is not treated soon enough.

Letter fluency   see *verbal fluency*

Levodopa   A precursor to dopamine, a neurotransmitter that is found at reduced levels in individuals with Parkinson's disease. Levodopa is used as a dopamine replacement agent for the treatment of Parkinson's disease. Unlike dopamine, levodopa can cross the blood–brain barrier where it is converted to dopamine.

Lewy body disease   A pathological condition caused by the accumulation of Lewy bodies (aggregations of alpha-synuclein protein) inside the nuclei of neurons in certain regions of the brain. Lewy body disease shares clinical and pathological features with Alzheimer's disease and Parkinson's disease. In dementia with Lewy bodies, deficits of attention, memory and executive function can be more severe than those found in Parkinson's disease dementia.

Lexeme   A semantic word. The lexeme is the basic unit of lexical semantics.

Lexical retrieval   The retrieval of words from a speaker's mental lexicon. Lexical retrieval is often impaired in people with aphasia and neurodegenerative disorders. It may manifest itself in the use of non-specific vocabulary (e.g. thing, stuff), the use of words that are semantically related to the target word (semantic paraphasias), or a tendency to 'talk around' a target word (circumlocution).

Lexical retrieval difficulty   see *anomia*

Lexical semantics   see *semantics*

Lexical substitution   A type of grammatical cohesion in which the substitute item and the item for which it substitutes have the same structural function. In the sentence *Mary bought* a house *and John sold* one, the word *one* has the function of a noun.

Linguistic competence   A native speaker's intuitive knowledge of the grammar of language, where 'grammar' is understood to include phonology, syntax and semantics. Chomsky distinguishes linguistic competence from performance.

Long Covid   The lack of recovery for several weeks or months following the start of symptoms that are suggestive of Covid infection, regardless of whether an individual has been tested or not.

Lower motor neuron   Neurons that transmit impulses for voluntary movement via spinal peripheral nerves or cranial nerves to skeletal muscles. Lower motor neuron lesions present with muscle atrophy, fasciculations (muscle twitching), decreased reflexes, decreased tone, negative Babinski sign and flaccid paralysis.

Lumbar puncture   Also known as a spinal tap, this procedure is undertaken to remove a small amount of cerebrospinal fluid from the spinal (vertebral) canal using a special needle. This fluid surrounds the brain and spinal cord. Its analysis can help in the diagnosis of infectious, degenerative, autoimmune and neoplastic conditions of the brain and spinal cord.

Magnetic resonance imaging (MRI)   A non-invasive imaging technology that produces three-dimensional anatomical images without the use of radiation. MRI can differentiate white matter from grey matter in the brain and can be used to diagnose tumours and aneurysms. When frequent imaging is required for diagnosis and therapy, it is the imaging method of choice owing to its lack of X-rays and other radiation.

Mania   Distinct periods of abnormally and persistently elevated, expansive or irritable mood. Mania is characterised by increased talkativeness, rapid speech, decreased need for sleep, racing thoughts, distractibility, increase in goal-directed activity and psychomotor agitation.

Memory   A higher-order cognitive function in which there is storage and recall of different types of information. Some forms of memory relate specifically to language (e.g. semantic memory), some are defined by temporal characteristics (e.g. short-term and long-term memory) and some contain personal life events (e.g. autobiographical memory). Injury and disease can disrupt specific types of memory. For example, impairment of episodic memory (i.e. recall of specific events) and working memory is a feature of Alzheimer's disease in the mild to moderate stages.

Meningitis   An inflammation of the protective membranes (meninges) that cover the brain and spinal cord. A bacterial or viral infection of the cerebrospinal fluid that surrounds the brain and spinal cord usually causes the inflammation. However, other types of infections, injuries, cancer and certain drugs can also cause meningitis.

Metaphor   A pragmatic phenomenon in which a speaker intends to describe an attribute of X by relating X to prominent features or characteristics of Y. For example, in the utterance *The rugby players were lions on the field*, a speaker does not intend to say that the players were actual lions, merely that the players were courageous, strong and fearless during a game of rugby.

Micrographia   Handwriting in Parkinson's disease may initially be of normal size but becomes progressively smaller, slower and more illegible as writing proceeds. Such 'slow' micrographia is distinguished from 'fast' micrographia, in which letters are small throughout and written at normal speed. The latter may occur in progressive supranuclear palsy.

Mild cognitive impairment   A condition in which individuals have more memory or other cognitive problems than is to be expected for their age, but their symptoms do not affect functioning. Mild cognitive impairment (MCI) has been described as pre-clinical Alzheimer's dementia (AD) as people with MCI can convert to AD. When memory is impaired, the condition is called 'amnestic MCI'. When non-memory cognitive domains such as language and executive function are impaired, the condition is called 'non-amnestic MCI'.

Miller-Fisher syndrome   see *Guillain-Barré syndrome*

Morphology   The linguistic discipline that studies the internal structure of words and the patterns and principles that underlie their composition. The morpheme is the unit of analysis.

Motor neurone disease   Also known as amyotrophic lateral sclerosis (US), motor neurone disease (MND) is a progressive neurodegenerative disease in which there is widespread and often rapid deterioration in upper and lower motor neurons. MND affects all aspects of speech production and eventually swallowing and feeding. There are four types of MND: amyotrophic lateral sclerosis (upper and lower motor neuron involvement); progressive bulbar palsy (upper and lower motor neuron involvement); progressive muscular atrophy (lower motor neuron involvement); and primary lateral sclerosis (upper motor neuron involvement).

Motor speech disorder   An impairment of speech production which may arise as a result of disruption in motor programming (apraxia of speech) and/or motor execution (dysarthria). Motor speech disorders may be developmental or acquired in nature and can result in mild to severe unintelligibility.

Motor speech production   The programming and execution of the motor processes that are required to produce speech. Motor speech production requires coordination of the following speech production sub-systems: articulation, resonation, phonation, respiration and prosody. Dysarthria and apraxia of speech are disorders of motor speech production.

Multiple sclerosis   An autoimmune disease in which there is demyelination of neurons in the central nervous system. There are three forms of MS: primary progressive, secondary progressive and relapsing-remitting. Dysarthria, dysphagia and cognitive impairment are present in a significant number of individuals with MS.

Multiple system atrophy A rare, progressive neurodegenerative disorder that is characterised by parkinsonism, cerebellar impairment and autonomic dysfunction. The pathological process in MSA is the deposition of aberrant α-synuclein protein in glia and neurons in multiple parts of the nervous system. The mean survival from time of diagnosis ranges from 6 to 10 years.

Mutation A permanent alteration in the DNA sequence that makes up a gene. A mutation can affect a single base pair or a large segment of a chromosome that includes multiple genes. Mutations can be hereditary (inherited from a parent) or somatic (present only in certain cells).

Myoclonus Sudden, involuntary jerking of a muscle or group of muscles. Myoclonus may occur in patients with multiple sclerosis, Parkinson's disease, Alzheimer's disease or Creutzfeldt-Jakob disease.

Narrative discourse A type of spoken or written discourse in which the events of a story are narrated to a listener or reader. The events so narrated are normally in the past and typically involve one or more actors.

Neologism This term literally means new ('neo') word ('logism'). Neologisms are often found in the expressive language of speakers with aphasia and dementia who have word-finding difficulties.

Neurodegenerative disorder A group of mainly age-dependent disorders with diverse pathophysiology and cognitive and motor symptoms. Common neurodegenerative disorders include Alzheimer's disease and Parkinson's disease.

Neuropsychiatric symptom Any one of the many behavioural symptoms that are associated with neurodegenerative disease. Neuropsychiatric symptoms include depression, anxiety, irritability and apathy. In more severe cases, these symptoms can take the form of aggression and hallucinations. Neuropsychiatric symptoms are associated with reduced quality of life and poor prognosis.

Noun phrase A noun and its pre-modifiers and post-modifiers. The pre-modifiers in a noun phrase include other nouns (e.g. brick *walls*) and adjectives (e.g. black *sheep*). The post-modifiers in a noun phrase include prepositional phrases (e.g. *students* in taxis), infinitives (e.g. *war* to end *all wars*) and relative clauses (e.g. *woman* who sings in the choir).

Nystagmus An involuntary, to-and-fro oscillation of the eyes that may be congenital or acquired and affect both eyes (bilateral) or only one eye (unilateral). Acquired nystagmus may be related to neurological disease (e.g. multiple sclerosis) or drug toxicity.

Obsessive compulsive disorder A neuropsychiatric disorder characterised by obsessions or compulsions (or both) that are distressing, time-consuming and cause substantial impairment. Obsessions are intrusive, unwanted thoughts (e.g. of contamination) that cause distress or anxiety. A person attempts to ignore or suppress obsessions with compulsions. Compulsions are repetitive behaviours or mental acts (e.g. washing) that the person feels compelled to perform in response to an obsession.

Oligoclonal bands   These are proteins called immunoglobulins. The presence of these proteins in the cerebrospinal fluid indicates inflammation of the central nervous system and may be used to make a diagnosis of multiple sclerosis.

Ophthalmoparesis/ophthalmoplegia   Weakness or paralysis of the extra-ocular muscles that control the movement of the eyes is called ophthalmoparesis and ophthalmoplegia, respectively. Cranial nerves III, IV or VI are usually involved. Ophthalmoparesis can be a symptom of many diseases (e.g. pituitary tumours) including neurogenerative disease.

Parietal lobe   The part of the cerebral cortex that lies between the occipital and frontal lobes, and above the temporal lobe. It processes sensory information for cognitive purposes and helps coordinate spatial relations.

Parkinson's disease   A neurodegenerative disease that is caused by the loss of cells that produce dopamine (a neurotransmitter substance) in the substantia nigra of the brain. The cardinal motor symptoms of Parkinson's disease are bradykinesia, tremor and rigidity. The most common form is idiopathic Parkinson's disease. Dysarthria and dysphagia are commonly seen in Parkinson's disease. Reduced vocal intensity (hypophonia) is an early feature of the disorder. Dementia can also occur in adults with Parkinson's disease.

Parkinson's plus syndrome   This refers to a group of neurodegenerative disorders that are characterised by features of Parkinson's disease but with other neurological symptoms or signs. They have a poor response to levodopa. Parkinson's plus syndrome includes progressive supranuclear palsy, multiple system atrophy and dementia with Lewy bodies.

Passive voice   Voice is a grammatical relationship between the subject and object in a sentence. In the active voice, the subject precedes the verb in the sentence (e.g. *Mary followed the man*). In the passive voice, the subject *Mary* follows the verb while the object *the man* precedes the verb (e.g. *The man was followed by Mary*). The three parts of the passive are part of the verb *be*, the passive participle and a *by* phrase. The *by* phrase is an optional element.

Past pointing test   In this test, the patient and examiner face each other. The examiner extends his arms and points straight ahead with index fingers 6 inches apart. The patient is asked to lift both arms overhead while pointing with both index fingers and then to bring down both arms and touch the examiner's index fingers while keeping arms extended. The process is repeated but this time with the patient keeping his eyes closed. In a positive test result, the patient's fingers will not line up to the examiner's fingers. This can indicate concussion or vestibular problems or injury to the cerebellum.

Patient   A semantic role that describes a person or thing that undergoes a process (e.g. The door opened).

Perseveration   The repetition of a linguistic form (word, phrase, etc.) beyond the point where it is appropriate. Perseveration is a feature of the spoken output of several types of clients with communication disorders, including adults with aphasia, patients with schizophrenia and clients with dementia.

Personal pronoun   see *pronoun*

Phenotype   The observable traits of an individual such as blood type, height and eye colour. The physical characteristics associated with the expression of genes.

Phonation   The production of voice by the laryngeal mechanism. Phonation is often impaired in speech disorders such as dysarthria. For example, weak, breathy phonation (hypophonia) is a feature of hypokinetic dysarthria in Parkinson's disease.

Phonemic cue   A prompt that may be used to elicit production of a target word and takes the form of the initial sound of the word, e.g. /s/ for 'sink'.

Phonemic fluency   see *verbal fluency*

Phonology   The study of the organisation of speech sounds into systems. Phonologists examine how sounds function contrastively to convey differences of meaning, e.g. a single phonetic difference of voicing between *pat* and *bat* conveys a difference of meaning. The phoneme is the unit of analysis.

Photophobia   This is defined as pain with normal or dim light. Photophobia is a common neurological and ophthalmological symptom and is associated with a range of conditions including migraine and traumatic brain injury.

Planning   Planning is a higher-order cognitive process that involves several aspects of executive function. These aspects include plan formulation, the monitoring and regulation of the responses to execute the plan, and the capacity to maintain goal representations in working memory.

Plantar reflex   This reflex is elicited by stroking the lateral part of the sole of the foot with a blunt object (e.g. end of a patella hammer). In a normal response, there is flexion of the big toe (hallux) with flexion and adduction of the other toes (so-called flexor plantar reflex). In an abnormal response, stroking produces extension (dorsiflexion) of the big toe with extension and abduction ('fanning') of the other toes (so-called extensor plantar reflex or Babinski reflex).

Pneumonia   An infection of the lungs that manifests in fever, cough and difficulty breathing. Pneumonia may be caused by bacteria, viruses and fungi, with some infections acquired in the community and others acquired in healthcare facilities. Pneumonia is a leading cause of death in people with neurodegenerative disorders where it is often associated with the entry of food and liquid into the lungs as a result of dysphagia (so-called aspiration pneumonia).

Positron emission tomography (PET)   This is a technique that measures physiological function by looking at blood flow, metabolism, neurotransmitters and radiolabelled drugs. PET is based on the detection of radioactivity emitted after a small amount of a radioactive tracer is injected into a peripheral vein. Among the many applications of this technique, PET can be used to track chemical neurotransmitters such as dopamine in Parkinson's disease.

Postural orthostatic tachycardia syndrome (POTS)   A group of symptoms that frequently occur when standing upright. In POTS, there is a heart rate increase from horizontal to standing of at least 30 beats per minute in adults (at least 40 beats per minute in adolescents), measured during the first 10 minutes of standing.

Pragmatics   The study of language use and aspects of meaning that are dependent on context. Pragmatic meaning is variously referred to as speaker meaning, implied meaning and non-literal meaning.

Preposition   A closed word class which occurs before a noun phrase (e.g. during *the cold weather*). Most prepositions are single words and are known as simple prepositions. Prepositions of more than one word are called complex prepositions and include two-word prepositions (e.g. *due to, along with*) and three-word prepositions (e.g. *in addition to*). Prepositions can express a range of meanings including space (e.g. next to *the church*), time (e.g. during *summer*) and means (e.g. with *an axe*). The term 'locative preposition' describes a preposition which expresses spatial meaning.

Presupposition   This describes information which is assumed, taken for granted or in the background of an utterance. Presuppositions reduce the amount of information that a speaker must explicitly state. They are triggered by certain lexical items (e.g. factive verbs *She* realised *the situation was hopeless*) and constructions (e.g. cleft construction It was *the boy who broke the window*).

Prevalence   The total number of individuals in a population who have a disease or health condition at a specific period of time. Prevalence is usually expressed as a percentage of the population.

Prognosis   The probability or risk of an individual developing a particular state of health (an outcome) over a specific period of time given that individual's clinical and non-clinical profile. An outcome may include an event such as death or a quantity such as disease progression.

Progressive aspect   Progressive aspect in English is encoded by the progressive auxiliary *be* followed by the *–ing* participle of a verb (e.g. *Jill is swimming; Frank was humming*). It indicates that an action or situation is ongoing.

Progressive non-fluent aphasia   Also known as non-fluent/agrammatic variant primary progressive aphasia (PPA), progressive non-fluent aphasia is one of the language variants of frontotemporal dementia. Clients with non-fluent/agrammatic variant PPA display grammatical simplification and errors in language production, effortful, halting speech with speech sound errors, impaired syntactic comprehension, spared content word comprehension and spared object knowledge.

Progressive supranuclear palsy A rare progressive neurological disorder with onset of symptoms after the age of 60 years. Clinical features include supranuclear vertical gaze palsy (difficulty shifting vertical gaze), frequent falls, bradykinesia (slowness of movement), axial (neck and trunk) rigidity, cognitive decline and communication impairments.

Pronominal reference The use of a pronoun to refer to a noun phrase. The noun phrase is called an 'antecedent'. In the sentence *Jackie bought a dress but then returned it to the shop*, the pronoun *it* refers to the noun phrase *a dress*.

Pronoun A closed word class that occurs in positions typically occupied by nouns (e.g. *Joan/she posted the parcel to the children/them*). Pronouns can be distinguished by case such as subject pronouns (e.g. *she, we*) and object pronouns (e.g. *her, them*). There are several different types of pronouns including personal pronouns (e.g. *I, you*), possessive pronouns (e.g. *my, our*), demonstrative pronouns (e.g. *this, those*), reflexive pronouns (e.g. *himself, ourselves*) and indefinite pronouns (e.g. *everything, somebody*).

Psychomotor slowing Also known as psychomotor retardation, this describes the slowing of motor and cognitive processes that is a feature of many neurodegenerative disorders, schizophrenia and depression. Psychomotor slowing affects speech, movement and ideation, and severely affects an individual's psychosocial functioning.

Psychomotor speed Psychomotor abilities relate to the relationship between cognitive functions and physical movements. Psychomotor speed can be calculated by examining an individual's ability to detect and respond to rapid changes in the environment, such as the presence of a stimulus.

Pyramidal sign A sign of damage to the pyramidal tract, a group of neurons that originate in the motor strip of the cortex and course downwards through the brain and into the spinal cord. Signs of pyramidal tract damage include weakness, spasticity, hyperreflexia, slowing of rapid alternating movements and a Babinski sign.

Rebound The rebound phenomenon is elicited by having a patient move a limb against resistance. When the resistance is suddenly removed, the limb normally moves a short distance in the desired direction and then rebounds (jerks back in the opposite direction). This phenomenon is present in normal limbs, exaggerated in spastic limbs and absent in limbs that are affected by cerebellar disease.

Reference The use of a linguistic expression to identify things in the external world. Reference is an important concept in a semantic account of meaning (hence, the term 'referential meaning').

Referent The object or event in the external world which is identified by an act of reference.

Relative clause A clause which modifies a noun, e.g. *the woman* <u>who bakes cakes</u>. Relative clauses are introduced by relative pronouns like *who, which, whom* and on occasion *that* (e.g. *This is the only house* <u>that is standing</u>).

REM sleep behaviour disorder Rapid eye movement (REM) sleep behaviour disorder is characterised by a loss of normal skeletal muscle atonia during REM sleep with prominent motor activity and dreaming. The emergence of REM sleep behaviour disorder in people over the age of 50 years has been suggested to be an early indicator of neurodegenerative diseases, including Parkinson's disease and Lewy body dementia.

Resonance see *resonation*

Resonation The vibrated airstream that is produced during phonation can assume a different timbre and intensity as it resonates in air-filled cavities in the pharynx, oral cavity and nasal cavities. Abnormal resonance can cause a voice disorder.

Respiration Inhalation and exhalation during breathing. Respiration is one of the speech production sub-systems. Impairments of respiration can lead to reduced breath support for speech in neurodegenerative diseases (e.g. motor neurone disease) and other conditions (e.g. cerebral palsy).

Retropulsion test Also known as the forced pull back test, this test assesses postural stability in patients with conditions such as Parkinson's disease. The patient is asked to stand with eyes open and feet comfortably apart. The examiner stands behind close to the patient and delivers a quick pull back on the patient's shoulders. The patient must maintain their stability and try not to move backwards. Patients with extrapyramidal disorders such as Parkinson's disease often show retropulsion and may take several steps backwards.

Rigidity Increased resistance during passive mobilisation of an extremity that is independent of direction and velocity of movement. Rigidity is one of the cardinal motor symptoms of Parkinson's disease.

Romberg test In this test, the patient stands with feet together, hands by the sides and eyes closed. With visual input cancelled, postural control relies on vestibular input and proprioceptive input alone. If a patient sways more than normal or falls without being held up by the examiner, the test is positive.

Saccade Rapid eye movements that are designed to shift the fovea (central region of the retina where vision is most acute) to objects of visual interest.

Semantic cue A prompt that describes some aspect of the meaning of a target word as a means of eliciting the word's production. For example, a semantic cue for the word 'lobster' might be *it lives in water and is a delicacy to eat*.

Semantic field A set of words that share a common semantic property. For example, 'guitar', 'flute', 'trumpet' and 'drum' all belong to the semantic field of musical instruments.

Semantic fluency see *verbal fluency*

Semantic paraphasia A language error in which a word that is semantically related to the target form is produced (e.g. 'ear' for *eye*). Semantic paraphasias are a feature of aphasia and language in dementia.

Semantic role   Semantic roles describe different entities in a situation and are associated with the argument structure of verbs, e.g. The flash of lightening$_{STIMULUS}$ blinded the onlookers$_{EXPERIENCER}$. Some semantic roles are obligatory in the argument structure of verbs and others are optional. For example, the agent is obligatory in the following sentence while the instrument is optional, e.g. The lorry driver$_{AGENT}$ stirred the coffee$_{PATIENT}$ with a spoon$_{INSTRUMENT}$.

Semantics   The study of the linguistic meaning of words (lexical semantics) and sentences.

Sjögren's syndrome   An autoimmune disease in which the immune system attacks the glands that make tears and saliva, causing dry eyes and a dry mouth.

Sleep apnoea   This disorder is characterised by frequent pauses in breathing during sleep usually accompanied by loud snoring. These pauses cut off oxygen supply to the body for a few seconds and the removal of carbon dioxide. The affected person wakes up, the airways are re-opened and breathing starts again. This cycle can happen repeatedly during the night, making proper sleep impossible and resulting in excessive daytime sleepiness.

Short-term memory   see *memory*

Social cognition   The cognitive capacity that allows us to attribute mental states to the minds of others. Also known as theory of mind, social cognition allows us to predict and explain the behaviour of others by means of establishing their cognitive (e.g. beliefs) and affective (e.g. sadness) mental states.

Spasticity   A condition in which the muscles are continuously contracted, causing muscle stiffness that can interfere with normal movement, speech and gait. Spasticity is a feature of many conditions including cerebral palsy, multiple sclerosis, traumatic brain injury and stroke.

Speech act   A term used by Austin and later Searle to describe utterances which perform acts or actions. Both Austin and Searle recognised different types of speech acts such as assertives (e.g. statements) and directives (e.g. requests).

Speech-language pathologist   The professional who assesses, diagnoses, and treats children and adults with communication and swallowing disorders. Speech-language pathologists are known as speech and language therapists in the UK and as logopaedists in some European countries.

Spinal cord   The major nerve tract of vertebrates that extends from the base of the brain through the spinal column. Its nerve fibres mediate reflex actions and transmit impulses to and from the brain. The spinal cord is covered by the same meninges that envelope the brain.

Spinal stenosis   This occurs when spaces in the spine narrow and create pressure on the spinal cord and nerve roots. Spinal stenosis occurs most often in the lower back (lumbar spinal stenosis) and the neck (cervical spinal stenosis).

Story grammar The structural components or elements that constitute a well-formed story, the way in which these components are arranged and the relationships among them. Most story grammars consist of an episode in a setting. The episode contains an event that brings about a reaction from the main character. This reaction leads the character to formulate a goal, make an attempt to reach the goal, achieve an outcome and arrive at an ending.

Stroke A stroke, or cerebrovascular accident, arises when there is disruption in the flow of blood through the vascular system of the brain. A stroke may be caused by a blood clot (embolus) in one of the blood vessels in the brain or leading to the brain (embolic stroke) or by a haemorrhage (haemorrhagic stroke) in one of these vessels.

Stuttering Also known as stammering; a fluency disorder which is characterised by word- and syllable-initial iterations (repetitions) and perseverations (prolongations). Stuttering occurs in developmental, acquired (mostly neurogenic) and psychogenic forms.

Subject A subject is a constituent that performs the action described by the predicate. In the sentence *Jack baked a cake*, the predicate (*baked a cake*) is performed by Jack. So, the noun phrase *Jack* is the subject of this sentence.

Subject complement A predicative complement which is co-referential with the subject in the sentence. The subject complement *teacher* is co-referential with the subject *Sally* in the sentence *Sally is a teacher*.

Subordinate clause see *subordinating conjunction*

Subordinating conjunction Conjunction words like *because, if* and *although* which link a dependent clause (a subordinate clause) to an independent clause (a main clause or sentence) are subordinating conjunctions. In the sentence *She missed school* <u>because she was ill</u>, the subordinating conjunction *because* introduces a subordinate clause which is dependent on the full sentence. Subordinating conjunctions can express a range of meanings. In the example just given, the subordinate clause expresses the reason why something happened (Why did she miss school? Reason: She was ill).

Subordination The use of subordinating conjunctions (e.g. *because, since*) or relative pronouns (e.g. *who, which*) to link clauses in such a way that one clause is dependent on (or subordinate to) another clause. In the following examples, the underlined clauses are subordinate to the main clause or sentence: Jack thought <u>that it must be Friday</u>; She enjoyed her job, <u>although she received a small salary</u>.

Substantia nigra (Latin: black substance) A long nucleus that is located in the midbrain. Functionally, it is considered to be a part of the basal ganglia because of its reciprocal connections with other brainstem nuclei. It consists of two components, the pars compacta and the pars reticulata. Degeneration of the pars compacta results in the reduced availability of the neurotransmitter dopamine in Parkinson's disease.

Suffix There are two types of suffixes in English words: inflectional suffixes and derivational suffixes. Inflectional suffixes have a grammatical function and include *–ed* to indicate past tense and *–ing* for progressive aspect. These suffixes create new word forms (not new words). Derivational suffixes are more numerous than inflectional suffixes. They change the class of words and in doing so create new words. For example, the suffix *–ion* changes *institute* from a verb to a noun (*institution*). In *fairness* and *agreement*, the suffixes *–ness* and *–ment* change an adjective and a verb, respectively, into nouns.

Superordinate term A word that names a general category and subsumes the meanings of other words within it. For example, *bird* is a superordinate of *eagle* and *parrot*.

Supraduction Upward movement of the eye. In a supraduction, the superior rectus muscle contracts and the inferior rectus muscle relaxes.

Supranuclear gaze palsy/paresis This is an impairment of horizontal gaze, vertical gaze or both. It results from dysfunction in the connections that are responsible for conducting voluntary gaze commands to the brainstem gaze centres. Vertical supranuclear gaze palsy is regarded as a cardinal visual feature of progressive supranuclear palsy.

Syntax The study of sentence structure. The aim of a syntactic analysis of a language is to produce a precise and rigorous description of the rules that characterise the phrases and sentences of that language. The ability to produce and understand syntactically well-formed sentences – expressive and receptive syntax, respectively – may be impaired in children and adults with language disorder.

Systematic review A review of all research studies and their findings relating to a particular question. The purpose of a systematic review is to identify all published and unpublished studies in an area, select those studies which satisfy certain criteria for inclusion, assess the quality of the studies and the evidence that they produce, synthesise their findings, and arrive at a balanced and impartial interpretation of their significance.

Tachycardia This refers to a rapid heartbeat of over 100 beats per minute. The consequences of tachycardia include chest pain, hypotension, and even cardiac arrest and death.

Tandem gait This is walking in which the heel of one foot is placed immediately in front of the toe of the other foot. It is used as a test of balance and coordination and is useful in identifying subtle or mild gait ataxia.

Tau pathology Tau is a protein that is associated with microtubules in a normal mature neuron. In Alzheimer's disease and related disorders called tauopathies, tau is abnormally hyperphosphorylated and accumulates as intraneuronal tangles.

Theory of mind The ability to attribute cognitive and affective mental states (e.g. beliefs, happiness) both to one's own mind and to the minds of others.

Deficits in theory of mind are a feature of many disorders in which there are significant communication problems including autism spectrum disorder, schizophrenia and dementia.

Tinnitus A roaring, buzzing or ringing sound in the ears which can impact on the mental health of affected individuals. Tinnitus is a symptom of many disorders including presbycusis, noise-induced hearing loss, ototoxicity related to the taking of aspirin and aminoglycoside antibiotics, Ménière's disease and acoustic neuroma.

Tonic-clonic seizure This type of seizure is characterised by clonic or myoclonic movements evolving to tonic muscle extension of the limb and trunk muscles followed by clonic contraction. Often these seizures are accompanied by biting of the tongue and urinary incontinence. Generalised tonic-clonic seizures are the most severe type of alcohol withdrawal seizures.

Tonsillectomy Surgical removal of the tonsils.

Topicalisation A syntactic movement in which a constituent is 'fronted', that is, placed at the beginning of a sentence, in order to give it prominence.

Topic management The selection, introduction, development and termination of a topic in conversation or other form of discourse. Topic management is disrupted in a range of clients with communication disorders, including individuals with autism spectrum disorder, schizophrenia, traumatic brain injury and dementia.

Transient ischaemic attack A transient ischaemic attack (TIA) is focal brain ischaemia that causes sudden, transient neurological deficits. TIAs are not accompanied by permanent brain infarction. Most TIAs are caused by emboli, usually from carotid or vertebral arteries.

Tremor One of the cardinal motor symptoms in Parkinson's disease. There are several different types of tremor in Parkinson's disease. However, the classic type is tremor-at-rest. As the name suggests, this tremor is seen at rest. However, in later stage disease, it may also occur in action, often with a short pause in the transition from rest to posture.

Traumatic brain injury An injury to the brain as a result of trauma sustained in a road traffic accident, trip or fall, violent assault, contact sport, or from a missile or projectile. There are two forms of traumatic brain injury (TBI). In an open or penetrating head injury, the skull is fractured or otherwise breached by a missile. In a closed head injury, the brain is damaged while the skull remains intact. TBI is a significant cause of death and disability in children and adults.

Turn taking The interactional nature of conversation is reflected in the exchange of turns between speaker and hearer. This two-way exchange of turns is known as turn taking. Turn taking is governed by rules about when it is appropriate to assume one's turn and relinquish it to another speaker.

Upper motor neuron   Nerves in the central nervous system that carry signals for voluntary movement. The primary tract that carries signals for voluntary movement is known as the pyramidal tract. The pyramidal tract further sub-divides into the corticospinal tract and the corticobulbar tract. Corticospinal tract fibres synapse with spinal nerves, while corticobulbar fibres synapse with cranial nerves. Upper motor neuron damage causes characteristic clinical symptoms including weakness, spasticity, clonus and hyperreflexia.

Utterance interpretation   The decoding of linguistic structures in an utterance sometimes arrives at the message that a speaker intended to convey. Often, however, an utterance must undergo further processing to arrive at a speaker's intended meaning. This additional processing, referred to as utterance interpretation, moves beyond rule-based processing of language to include inferences about a speaker's communicative intention.

Verb phrase   A verb and its pre-modifiers and post-modifiers. Auxiliary verbs (e.g. has been *waiting*), negative forms (e.g. never *cleans*), and adverbs (e.g. purposefully *hid*) can be pre-modifiers in verb phrases. Post-modifiers in verb phrases include noun phrases (e.g. *stole* the ornament), adjectives (e.g. *became* angry), adverbs (e.g. *walked* slowly), prepositions (e.g. *stood* next to *the pillar*) and clauses (e.g. *hoped* that she would leave).

Verbal fluency   A cognitive-linguistic skill that involves access to the mental lexicon and executive control. Verbal fluency is included in a neuropsychological assessment and is tested by means of phonemic (letter) fluency tasks and semantic (category) fluency tasks. In letter fluency tasks, the patient is asked to recall as many words as possible beginning with a certain letter (usually 'F') in one minute. In category fluency tasks, the patient is asked to name as many words as possible belonging to a particular semantic field (usually animals) in one minute. Norms for both letter and category fluency are now available.

Visual perception   The recognition of visual information that arrives in the brain from the peripheral organs of vision, namely, the eyes. Visual agnosia occurs when the brain cannot recognise the visual information that it receives from the eyes.

Vital capacity   This refers to the maximal volume of air that can be expired following maximum inspiration.

Vocabulary   The words of a language, sometimes called the lexicon. Lexicology is the branch of linguistics that studies the vocabulary of a language. A speaker's expressive vocabulary is the words that he can produce. Receptive vocabulary describes the words that a speaker can understand. Expressive and receptive vocabulary may be reduced in adults with neurodegenerative disorders.

Voice disorder   Also called 'dysphonia', a voice disorder may be organic (i.e. have a structural or neurological aetiology) or functional in nature (i.e. have a psychogenic or hyperfunctional aetiology). Regardless of aetiology, the effect of a voice disorder on the perceptual attributes of the voice may be captured by terms such as 'hoarse', 'breathy', and 'strained-strangled'.

Voice quality   The quality of a speaker's voice is a multidimensional concept that has perceptual, acoustic and physiological components. Voice quality is often captured by terms like 'breathy', 'hoarse' and 'strained-strangled'.

Wernicke's encephalopathy   An acute neurological condition characterised by a clinical triad of ophthalmoparesis with nystagmus, ataxia and confusion. It is caused by thiamine deficiency in people with long-term alcohol abuse. Wernicke's encephalopathy (WE) is differentiated from Korsakoff's syndrome, a neuropsychiatric disorder that is a consequence of at least one episode of WE.

Word-finding difficulty   see *anomia*

Working memory   see *memory*

References

[1] Hu, M.T.M., Ellis, C.M., Al-Chalabi, A., Leigh, P.N. and Shaw, C.E. (1998) 'Flail arm syndrome: A distinctive variant of amyotrophic lateral sclerosis', *Journal of Neurology, Neurosurgery & Psychiatry*, 65 (6): 950–951.

[2] Hübers, A., Hildebrandt, V., Petri, S., Kollewe, K., Hermann, A., Storch, A., Hanisch, F., Zierz, S., Rosenbohm, A., Ludolph, A.C. and Dorst, J. (2016) 'Clinical features and differential diagnosis of flail arm syndrome', *Journal of Neurology*, 263: 390–395.

APPENDIX

Sam and Fred Story (Immediate and Delayed Recall)

A short story was read aloud to participants who were then asked to recall it. The story captured a plausible scenario and used familiar vocabulary. It contained 104 words in total. There were eight sentences, ranging in length from five words to 16 words. The average sentence length was 13 words. The same verbal instruction was given to all participants: "I'm going to tell you a short story. I want you to listen to it carefully. I will then ask you to tell it back to me".

Sam and Fred were brothers who had farmed the same land for thirty years. They had been closely following weather forecasts and knew that the weather was about to change. They had been working frantically in the fields when suddenly the skies opened. Several days of hard labour were disappearing before their eyes as crops were washed away. To add to their difficulties, the storm ripped open the door of the barn. Many sheep and cows escaped. People from the local village arrived to help the two distressed farmers. It was nearly nightfall by the time all the animals were returned to the barn.

Cookie Theft Picture Description Task

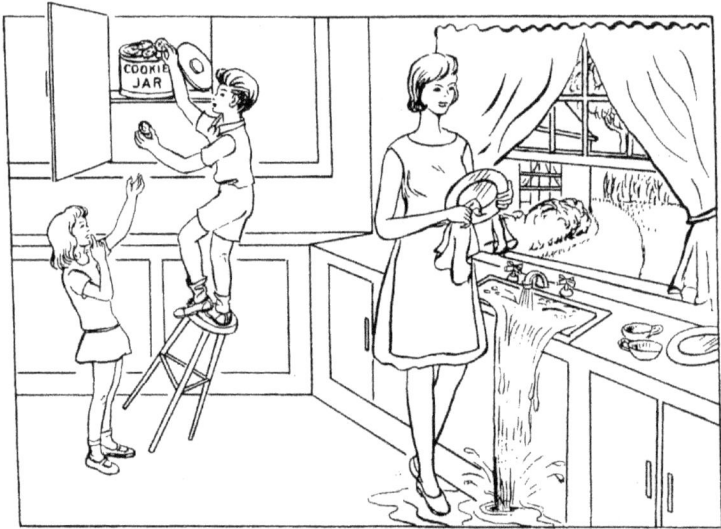

FIGURE A.1 Cookie Theft picture (reproduced from H. Goodglass, E. Kaplan and B. Barresi (2001) *Boston Diagnostic Aphasia Examination*, Third Edition *(BDAE-3)*, Austin, TX: PRO-ED; Used with permission of PRO-ED, Inc.)

Flowerpot Incident Narrative

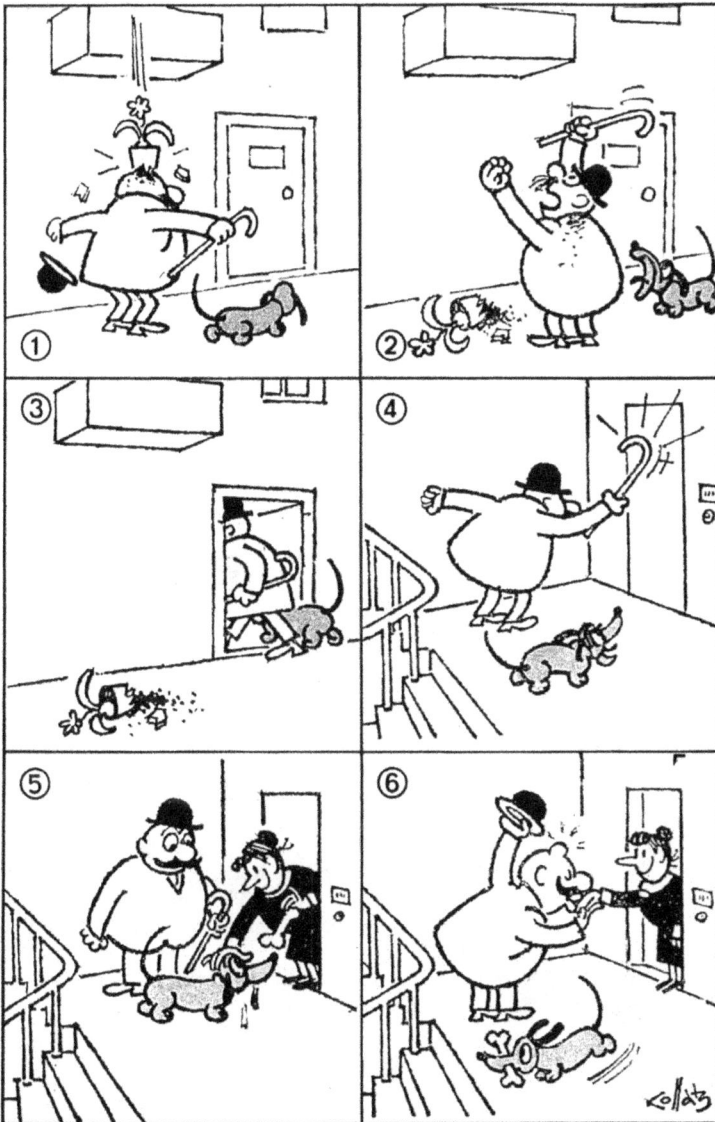

FIGURE A.2 Flowerpot Incident stimulus (from I. Schüßler and R. Tzschoppe (1972) *So ein Dackel! 22 Bildgeschichten für den Sprachunterricht*, Illustrator H. Kossatz, Stuttgart: Ernst Klett Verlag)

INDEX

Page numbers in **bold** indicate tables.

adductor jerk 118
adverb 34, 46, 50, 106, 184
aetiology 4
affective mental state 18, 35, 51, 72, 163,
    167, 183, 188, 199
agent 31, 70–71, 86, 88, 105, 122, 139, 182
aggression 134
agrammatism 7, 12; *see also* aphasia
akinesia 6
alcohol-related brain damage 133
Alzheimer's: dementia 61; disease 10, 25, 46,
    98, 196; pathology 6; *see also* dementia
amyotrophic lateral sclerosis (ALS)
    117–118, 125; *see also* motor neurone
    disease
anaphoric reference 73–74, 89–90, 93,
    107, 125, 164, 184, 187; *see also*
    cataphoric reference
antidepressant 8
anxiety 42, **64**, 99, 118
apathy 42, 134
aphasia 7, 25, 201
apomorphine 100–101
apraxia 6
apraxia of speech 25, 92, 102, 110, 121,
    126, 136, 159, 166, 179
argument structure 160, 166
arrhythmia 174
articulation 35, 45, 52, 85, 110, 126, 136,
    166, 179, 186

aspiration pneumonia 42
ataxia 62, 134, 172, 174
atrophy 9, 135
attention 8, 42, **64**, 65, 100, 119, 144, 156,
    162–167, 175, **176**, 177, 188, 197
augmentative and alternative
    communication (AAC) 118
autonomic disease/disorder 99, 118, 172
axial rigidity 24
axon 82, 172

bradykinesia 24, 60, 63, 99
brainstem 25
breathing 35, 61–62, 102, 126, 157, 175
bulbar symptom 24, 118

cataphoric reference 107; *see also*
    anaphoric reference
category fluency 45, 70, 75, 88, 139, 161,
    180–181, 187, 196; *see also* semantic
    fluency
central nervous system 82
cerebellar sign 62–63
cerebrospinal fluid 62
cholecystectomy 156
Chomsky, Noam 201
chorea 42
chronic fatigue syndrome 159, 163
circumlocution 19, 177, 180, 187, 200
cirrhosis 135, 143

clause 29–30, 46–47, 69, 103, 121–122, 137, 159–160, 180

clonus 62

cognition 19, 36, 53, 65, 76, 93, 111, 126, 137, 147–148, 159, 167, 175, 185, 187, 202

cogwheeling 62

cohesion 15, 34, 50, 107, 124, 141–142, 164, 167, 198, 201–202

cohesive device 16, 125

communicative: competence 194, 201–202; intention 198, 201

compensation 200

comprehensibility 184

comprehension 7, 11–12, 19, 25, 31, 45–46, 49, 52, 69, 71, 87, 89, 104–106, 110, 121, 137, 160, 166, 179, 182, 186–187, 196, 200

computerized axial tomography (CAT or CT scan) 7, 62–63

confrontation naming 9, **11**, **14**, 30–31, 36, 47–48, 76, 92, 104, 110, 121–122, 126, 137, 140, 145, 148, 161, 166, 177, 180–181, 187, 195, 201–202

conjunctivitis 157, 175

content word 15, 87, 196

conversational: discourse 184; exchange 33, 202; partner 194, 200, 202; repair 35–36, 50, 53, 76, 89, 92, 106, 110, 201

corticobasal degeneration 6

coughing 157, 175

cranial nerve 172

cueing 195, 201, 203

deictic expression 49, 124, 164–165

deixis 34, 36, 49–50, 53, 71, 76, 89, 92, 106, 110, 124, 126, 165–166, 183, 187, 201

delirium 64

delusion 60, 64

dementia: with Lewy bodies 1, 60–61, 67, 73, 198; Parkinson's disease 67

demonstrative pronoun 34, 49, 125, 141, 184

demyelination 82; see also multiple sclerosis

depression 60, **64**, 65, 84, 99, 101, 118–119, 134

depth perception 175

derivational morphology 36, 86

derivational suffix 29, 46, 137, 159

dialect 86

diplopia 26

direct reported speech 74, 76, 90, 92, 124, 126, 165, 167

dopamine 60, 63, 98; see also Parkinson's disease

drooling 9

duopa 100–101

dysarthria 28, 44, 52, 67, 83, 85, 92, 102, 121, 126, 136, 159, 166, 179

dysfluency 12, 68

dyskinesia 100

dysphagia 24, 83, 118

dysphoria 42

dystonia 6, 42

ellipsis 19, 34, 36, 50, 53, 73–74, 89, 93, 107, 141, 148, 164, 166, 184, 187, 198

emotion 52, 177

Epstein-Barr virus 82, 173

executive: dysfunction 88, 93, 105, 111, 198; function 7–8, 13, 19, 36, 42, 45, 53, 104, 123, 126, 137, 139, 144, 148, 156, 162–163, 165, 167, 177–178, 186, 197–198

facial expression 7, 9, 25–26, 36, 72, 99, 102, 111, 120, 185

fasciculation 118

figurative language 49, 71, 76, 126, 199

filler 19, 87, 93, 161, 165, 180, 196

flail arm syndrome 118

fluency 12, 31, 35, 45, 52, 65, 67–68, 75, 86, 102, 121, 126, 166

gastroesophageal reflux 178

gastroparesis 175

gesture 9, **14**, 18, 36, 44, 72, 102, 111, 120, 164, 199–200

grammar 52, 69, 201

gross motor movement 9

Guillain-Barré syndrome 172, 184, 197

hallucination 60, **64**, 66, 68

hedging 91–92, 182, 187

humour **11**, 15, 19, 36, 50, 53, 71–72, 76, 140, 148, 187; see also joke

Huntington's disease 42

hyperbole 71, 88, 92, 123–124, 126

hypernasality 45

hypertension 27, 155–156, 158

hypokinetic dysarthria 28, 102

hypometabolism 9

hypomimia 62

idiom 15, 19, 49, 53, 71–72, 76, 88–89, 92, 123, 126, 183, 187, 202

impulsivity **11**, 26, 36

incidence 6, 24, 42, 60, 98, 172
inference 16, 19, 73, 89–90, 92, 125–126, 129, 142–143, 146–148, 198, 201–202
infinitive clause 29, 46, 52, 69, 86, 103, 137, 180, 195
inflectional morphology 19, 29, 36, 52, 76, 86, 102–103, 110, 121, 137, 148, 179
inflectional suffix 46, 68–69, 137, 159, 166, 179, 186–187
information: management 33, 107–108, 111; processing 8, 53, 86–87, 161, 165, 187
informativeness 162, 165–166, 185
inhibition 13, 177, 186, 188
instrument 31, 139
intellectual function 8
intelligibility 19, 28, 35, 45, 52, 75, 92, 102, 110, 126, 148, 166, 186
intention tremor 62
intonation 10, 19, 35, 44, 52, 67, 86, 102, 110, 121, 126, 137, 159, 166
irony 106
ischaemia 7

joke 8; *see also* humour

keratoconus 174
knee jerk reflex 118
Korsakoff's syndrome 133; *see also* alcohol-related brain damage

language: expressive 12, 36, 45, 86, 102, 105, 110, 121, 123, 126, 138, 148, 159, 161, 166, 183; receptive 36, 121; written 179
lesion 84, 135, 143
letter fluency 31, 45, 67, 70, 88, 93, 105, 123, 137, 139, 162, 165, 167, 185–186, 188, 198; *see also* phonemic fluency
levodopa 10, 27
Lewy body disease 60–61, 69, 73, 98, 198
lexeme 161
lexical: reiteration 107, 164, 166; retrieval 13–14, 19, 28–30, 45, 87–88, 93, 104–105, 139, 145, 161, 181, 195–196, 201; semantics 139, 201; substitution 16, 19, 73–74, 93, 124, 126, 141, 148, 164, 166, 184
linguistic competence 194, 201–202
long Covid 157, 159, 163, 178
lower motor neuron 117
lumbar puncture 62, 119, 175

magnetic resonance imaging (MRI) 7, 9, 83–84, 99, 119, 175
mania 65

memory: long-term 84; short-term 8–9, 26, 84, 178; verbal 8, 65, 76, 142, 176; working 8, 32, 84, 110, 160, 175
meningitis 62
mental health 157
mental state: attribution 72, 76, 125, 147, 163, 183, 188, 199; language 19, 35–36, 51, 53, 92, 111, 126, 183, 199; *see also* theory of mind
metaphor 71, 88–89, 92, 110
micrographia 63
mild cognitive impairment 104, 135, 144, 148, 176
Miller-Fisher syndrome 172–173, 175–176, 178–179; *see also* Guillain-Barré syndrome
motor neurone disease (MND) 117–126, 196–200, 203; *see also* amyotrophic lateral sclerosis
motor speech disorder 7, 75, 92, 148, 179, 186
motor speech production 102
multiple sclerosis (MS) 82–92, 198
mutation 45
myoclonus 6, 60

narrative: discourse 198; fictional 146, 162; production 15, 92
nasal resonance 45
neologism 196
neurodegenerative: disease 42, 53; disorder 86, 92, 98
neurologist 7, 9–10, 20, 25, 43, 61–63, 65–66, 84, 87, 99–100, 118–119, 183
neurology 83, 100
neuron 24, 60, 117
neuropsychiatric symptom 42, 99, 118, 177–178
neuropsychologist 9
non-literal language 71, 88, 92
noun phrase 161, 165
nystagmus 134

occupational: exposure 117; functioning 85; therapy 10, 26, 43, 119, 175
oligoclonal bands 62
ophthalmoparesis/ophthalmoplegia 24, 134, 172

paralysis 83, 188
parietal lobe 9
Parkinson's disease (PD) 7, 10, 25–27, 61, 63, 67, 98–102, 104, 106–107, 110–112, 118, 122, 198–200, 203
Parkinson's plus syndrome 63

passive voice 29, 46, 52, 103, 110, 122, 126, 159–160, 166, 180, 187, 195
past pointing test 62
pause 15
peripheral nervous system 62
perseveration 17, 45, 48, 52
personal pronoun 102, 125
phenotype 6–7, 82
phonation 186
phonemic: cue **14**, 30, 47, 70, 104, 110, 138, 145, 195; fluency 13, 19, 29, 31, 36, 45, 53, 76, 88, 104–105, 111, 122–123, 126, 137, 139, 144, 148, 197; see also letter fluency
phonology 45, 52, 148, 201
photophobia 175
planning 19, 28, 44, 47, 53, 69, 87, 104, 119, 126, 197
plantar reflex 62, 118
pneumonia 42, 61, 173
pointing 62, 200
politeness 166
postural orthostatic tachycardia syndrome (POTS) 174
pragmatic language skill 35, 72, 76, 88, 123, 126, 141–142, 182, 184, 187
pragmatics 15–16, 19, 31, 36, 50, 53, 71, 73, 76, 88, 92, 106, 110, 126, 140, 148, 164, 166, 183, 187, 195, 201–202
preposition 49, 52, 139
presupposition 34–35, 52–53, 71, 76, 126, 164–166, 183, 201
prevalence 6, 24, 42, 60, 82, 84, 98, 117, 133
procedural discourse 50, 166
prognosis 119
progressive aspect 29, 180
progressive non-fluent aphasia 7, 25
progressive supranuclear palsy 24; see also Parkinson's disease
pronominal reference 16, 34, 36, 53, 142, 148, 198
pronoun 16, 19, 50–51, 53, 72, 138, 141–142, 163, 165, 200
prosody 45, 179
proverb 71
psychomotor speed 42
pyramidal sign 63

quality of life 83, 203

reasoning 64
rebound 62
referent 16, 19, 51, 53, 141, 164
rehabilitation 10

relative clause 29–30, 46, 52, 69, 87, 103, 121–122, 126, 137, 160, 195
REM sleep behaviour disorder 60, 63, **64**, 66
reported speech 184, 187
resonance 45, 67, 86, 102, 121, 128, 136, 159, 179, 186
retropulsion test 63
rigidity 6, 60, 63, 99
Romberg test 62

saccade 175
script 90–93, 109
seizure 60, 134, 143–144
semantic: cue **14**, 47–48, 87, 104, 110, 122, 138, 145, 195; field 138, 145; fluency **11**, 13, 19, 25, 31, 36, 45, 52, 88, 92, 105, 110, 122, 126, 139, 144–145, 166; role 31, 36, 70, 76, 92, 105, 110, 123, 126, 160, 182, 187
semantics 19, 36, 49, 52, 76, 88, 92, 110, 126, 148, 160, 166, 181, 187, 201–202
Sjögren's syndrome 174
sleep apnoea 62
social: cognition 147, 198; interaction 179; relationship 135
spasticity 83
speech act 105–106
speech and language therapy 10, 27, 53, 102, 119
speech-language pathologist 201
speech production 28, 44, 67, 75, 92, 102, 110, 120
spinal cord 117
spinal stenosis 62, 67
story: grammar 91–92, 126, 198, 202; telling 17, 51, 89–90, 162, 197–198
striatum 46
stroke 26
stuttering 8
subject complement 46
subordinate clause 29–30, 47, 69, 87, 103, 121, 126, 137, 160, 180
subordinating conjunction 49, 52
subordination 12
substantia nigra 98; see also Parkinson's disease
supraduction 175
supranuclear gaze palsy/paresis 8
swallowing 26–27, 50, 61, 83, 101, 119, 173–174, 184
syntax 12, 19, 29–30, 36, 46, 52, 76, 86–88, 92, 103
systematic review 60, 156

tachycardia 174–175, 184
tandem gait 62
tau pathology 6
theory of mind (TOM) 18–19, 35–36, 51,
    53, 72, 76, 106, 111, 125, 141, 163,
    182–183, 188, 198
tinnitus 175
tonic-clonic seizure 143
tonsillectomy 156
topic: digression 71, 198; management 15,
    148
topicalisation 46, 52, 195, 201
tremor 9, 60, 62–63, **64**, 99, 177
turn taking 15, 89, 148

upper motor neuron 117
utterance interpretation 183, 198

verbal fluency 8–9, 42, 65, 76, 88, 177
verb phrase 47, 69
vision 26, 63, **64**, 83–84, 99, 156, 175
visual: hallucination 60, 64; impairment
    120, 177, 185; perception 64
vital capacity 119
vocabulary 19, 36, 52, 76, 92, 110, 126,
    148, 166, 180, 187
vocal volume 19, 121, 159
voice quality 44, 52, 67, 86, 102, 121, 126,
    137, 159, 166, 179

Wernicke's encephalopathy 133–134
word-finding difficulty 8–9, 14–15, 19, 31,
    36, 52, 76, 87, 92, 105, 110, 122, 139,
    148, 161, 166, 181, 196, 200, 202–203
writing 63, 66–67, 74, 163

For Product Safety Concerns and Information please contact our EU
representative GPSR@taylorandfrancis.com
Taylor & Francis Verlag GmbH, Kaufingerstraße 24, 80331 München, Germany

www.ingramcontent.com/pod-product-compliance
Lightning Source LLC
Chambersburg PA
CBHW060252220326
41598CB00027B/4069

*9 7 8 0 3 6 7 7 2 1 3 0 5 *